Nurse–Social Worker Collaboration in Managed Care

Joellen Hawkins, RNC, PhD, FAAN, began her love affair with settlement houses and became interested in the collaboration between nurses and social workers because of the stories her Aunt Tommy told of her work as a public health nurse in Chicago in the 1920s. Formally Lillian Beck Fuller, Aunt Tommy was first assigned to the Hull-House station of the Chicago VNA and remembered having lunch with Jane Addams and being part of the work of the settlement house. Joellen Hawkins is a Professor in the School of Nursing at Boston College and has authored more than 2 dozen books and over 100 articles. The history of nurses, nursing, and of women as caregivers is her avocation. Her current work includes an historical investigation of the often hidden roles of women in the settlement house movement.

Nancy Veeder, MSW, MBA, PhD, has been engaged in health and mental health services delivery and research in the United States, Jamaica, and Mauritus, Indian Ocean. Interdisciplinary collaboration played out in community settings, especially that between the historical allies social work and nursing, has been a major focus of her practice, research, and writing. Dr. Veeder is an Associate Professor at Boston College Graduate School of Social Work, where she teaches research and management. Her two other books are on women's decision making and human services marketing.

Carole Pearce, RNC, PhD, is an Assistant Professor in the Department of Nursing, College of Health Professions, University of Massachusetts—Lowell where she teaches graduate students in the family and community nurse practitioner program. Her areas of interest include women's health, managed care, culture, and nursing theory. As a nurse practitioner, she maintains a practice in an inner-city women's health care center and focuses her current research on pregnancy and prenatal care with an emphasis on Hispanic women, pregnancy outcomes, and domestic violence. Publications to date concentrate on pregnancy, prenatal care, and curriculum changes.

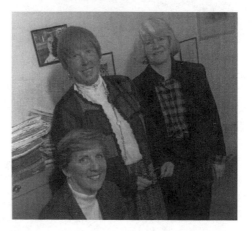

Prof. Carole W. Pearce, Prof. Nancy Veeder, and Prof. Joellen Hawkins, from left.

Nurse–Social Worker Collaboration in Managed Care

A Model of Community Case Management

Joellen W. Hawkins
RNC, PhD, FAAN

Nancy W. Veeder
MSW, MBA, PhD

Carole W. Pearce
RNC, PhD

 Springer Publishing Company

Springer Publishing Company, Inc.
536 Broadway
New York, NY 10012-3955

Cover design by Margaret Dunin
Acquisitions Editor: Ruth Chasek
Production Editor: Pamela Lankas

98 99 00 01 02 / 5 4 3 2 1

Library of Congress Cataloging-in-Publication Data

Hawkins, Joellen Watson.
    Nurse–social worker collaboration in managed care : a model of community
case management / Joellen W. Hawkins, Nancy W. Veeder, Carole W. Pearce.
        p.   cm.
    Includes bibliographical references and index.
    ISBN 0-8261-9830-9
    1. Primary nursing.   2. Medical social work.   3. Managed care plans
(Medical care)   I. Veeder, Nancy W.   II. Pearce, Carole W.   III. Title.
    RT90.7.H39   1997
    610.73—dc21
                                                                    97-22490
                                                                    CIP

Printed in the United States of America

Contents

Foreword

Nurses and social workers have been partners in care for so many years that it may seem to them that collaboration is both obvious and easily accomplished. As more and more care has moved from acute settings into community-based practice, nurses and social workers are struggling to help patients and families gain the equilibrium and skill it takes to become managers of their own care. It is not an easy task. Further, the financial chaos now present in the health care system sets the stage for competition among providers, gaps in essential care, and changes in both the technical and social support systems patients and their families have come to depend on.

The tensions and conundrums created by the managed care era of the late 20th century puts the public in many difficult positions. They must choose among providers without real knowledge of how their roles should be combined. They have limited resources to pay them and new choices to make about what kind of care they need. They find themselves with new power, but little education about how to manage an unwieldy health care system. Providers are also in turmoil. They are confused and worried about themselves and their patients. They are working in new and often different physical settings where change is the constant, and rules that have long applied, no longer do. Their education may no longer serve them well, and the opportunity to advance in their careers may be curtailed. All of these observations may cast an inordinately gloomy perspective on the future of health care in our country. The climate may appear to be totally inhospitable to collaborative efforts that require a modicum of harmony, mutual cooperation and respect, and mental freedom to experiment with new ideas. But, it is the perfect time for collaborative efforts among providers, patients, families, and communities. Collaboration can bring chaos to its knees, bring out the brightest and newest approaches to problem solving, and build new bridges of cooperation over long-standing rifts. This is the preferable scenario for our times. Certainly nurses and social workers will be powerful brokers and major resources in bringing useful, lasting, and flexible change to health care in the future.

Collaborative work is not easy. The literature about collaboration is uneven, with the majority of collaborative models presented in the 1970s and 1980s. Most of this work describes relationships between physicians and nurses. To study collaboration it is necessary to look at the elements of structure, process and outcome, as well as interpersonal relationships. Effective collaborative practices require that skilled individuals, with differing areas of expertise work together in a fluid, reciprocal fashion. There needs to be both assertive and cooperative behavior. The collaborators must be able to provide a new kind of care that results from the combination of unique skills (Siegler & Whitney, 1994).

Nurses and social workers are now warned by both insiders and outsiders that they are treading on each other's territory, and they had best beware lest one take the other's "territory" away. Yet, historically, these two sets of professionals have always worked together, and no where more effectively than in the community. Now, we are faced with health care models that are increasingly more community based. It is an arena ripe for the collaboration of all professionals. More to the point, it is an opportunity for reintroducing the effective, complementary work of nurses and social workers that marked the early years of the 20th century and laid the groundwork for the social revolution that improved the public health of our nation immeasurably.

It is in times of great change that the most innovative and useful models can be introduced and tested. Joellen Hawkins, Nancy Veeder, and Carole Pearce have based their timely book, *Nurse–Social Worker Collaboration in Managed Care,* on a qualitative research project among nurses and social workers that resulted in the development of a collaborative model of cooperation between the two professions. The Biopsychosocial Individual and Systems Intervention Model (BISIM) introduced in the book gives form and framework to collaboration between nurses and social workers in an era of managed care that is both useful and concrete. Its structure is based on a client/system focus, using a transdisciplinary case-management approach by advanced practitioner teams. It is a flexible, community-based approach with a strong advocacy focus throughout the life span. It mobilizes the client competencies, and uses a community-health education/physical-and-mental-illness-prevention basis for care. It involves continual assessment of community needs, as well as those of individuals, groups, communities, and organizations. It is based on the known components needed for collaborative practice. At the heart of it is mutual respect for unique and shared skills between nurses and social workers, commitment to seamless care trajectories, accountability, and quality assurance for outcomes.

The authors have provided information about managed care, the histori-cal background for nurse–social work collaboration, current concerns and conundrums, and the role of other disciplines in the collaborative effort. Contributors have added sections related to implementing the BISIM in the community, models of hospital-based care, existing community mod-els, and physician roles in managed care. The Appendix includes the study design for the qualitative study that underpins the model.

This book will be useful to students and practitioners in collaborative efforts. More, it is a tribute to the long, mutually satisfying relationships nurses and social workers have had in caring together for people. For those of us who have come to expect that these two professions work together, it heightens the awareness of problems that need to be faced if we are to continue in the same fashion in the future. Perhaps the most important contribution it makes is to reaffirm the basic decency of our work together. It proposes we have a mutual understanding that patients and their families need coaches in their quest to comprehend and use a new and evolving health care system, and that together, we are the key to a winning team.

FAY W. WHITNEY, PHD, RN, FAAN
Professor
University of Wyoming
School of Nursing
Laramie, WY

REFERENCE

Siegler, E. L., & Whitney, F. W. (1994). *Nurse–physician collaboration: Care of adults and the elderly* (pp. 3–8). New York: Springer Publishing Co.

Foreword

In 1905 Ida Maud Cannon, a nurse who was influenced by Jane Addams to also become a social worker, began with Dr. Richard Cabot the first organized social work effort in a hospital-based clinic. They asked, "Why do so many cases of tuberculosis come to us from localities where factories and quarries furnish employment for most of the working people? Why is a certain town sending us so many unmarried pregnant girls? How does it happen that another patient is suffering from lead poisoning after 1 month's employment in a storage-battery factory?" In their quest to "make medical care effective" and "cure consumption" they enlisted social workers, nurses, physicians, and volunteers (Massachusetts General Hospital, 1905–1915).

As an inheritor of this legacy of strong discipline-specific education combined with collaborative practice, I was honored to participate in the study on which this book is based, but skeptical about its outcome. Believing in collaboration (why else would I practice in an interdisciplinary setting) but committed to a discipline (social work), managing both interdisciplinary programs (Family Care; Domestic Violence) and a social work department, I questioned how this book would inform, challenge, and support what was, is, and could be.

This book practices what it preaches—collaboration. it brings together what is best in academia with what is best in practice. While highlighting history enough to inform (even surprise), it documents what is current (well known and little known). Building on the strengths and limitations of two disciplines, it supports and challenges while recommending a forward-thinking practice model.

In this era of health and human services that advertise cost-effectiveness but fund the least expensive option, that celebrates diversity but sells one-size-fits-all, and that promotes collaboration but rewards competition, this book is straightforward, thought provoking, and action enabling.

EVELYN E. BONANDER, MSW
Director of Social Services
Massachusetts General Hospital
Boston, MA

REFERENCE

Massachusetts General Hospital. (1905–1915). *Reports of the Social Service Department.* Boston, MA: Author.

Acknowledgments

Collaboration is a complex process involving communication, mutual respect, tolerance, flexibility, focus, shared goals, forthrightness, self-confidence about one's knowledge and skills, sensitivity, and above all else, humor. In addition, interdisciplinary collaboration combines the best of several worlds. The social work–nurse collaborative team model proposed in this book embodies all of these. This point became evident during the writing of this book when we realized that we were actually employing the interdisciplinary collaborative model we were proposing. That the model worked so well in practice was intellectually rewarding. That it was such fun in the implementation was a wonderful personal dividend for each of us.

So many people deserve our gratitude. The librarians are first. Without these dedicated and knowledgeable people on the team, no academic undertaking will succeed. We are especially grateful to librarians at the O'Neill and Graduate School of Social Work Libraries at Boston College and O'Leary Library at the University of Massachusetts—Lowell (both the interlibrary loan and circulation desks).

Next come our students, who are delightfully inquisitive and supportive of our projects, asking the most incisive questions, which never fail to keep us on our toes. If they don't get it, it isn't to be gotten.

And finally our thanks go to those students—Valerie Hamel, Carol McMahon-Morin, and Ellen Trabka—who assisted us in interviewing participants in the study reported in this book, and who wrote or assisted in writing chapters 9, 10, and 11. These individuals both broadened and deepened our perspectives immeasurably. Susan Williams, coauthor of chapter 7 and a supervisor of both social workers and nurses in a community health and behavioral health setting, provided rare insights and current practice examples that could only be offered by someone who is both a registered nurse and a social worker.

We especially wish to thank each of the nurse and social work participants who were so generous, insightful, and conceptually clear in the interviews they gave for our study. These leaders in the health field formed the core practice insights for this book. They are:

Susan S. Bailis, MSW
Shelley L. Baranowski, RN, MS
Evelyn E. Bonander, ACSW
Don Bowdoin, LICSW
Joyce C. Clifford, RN, MSN, FAAN
Jeanette G. Clough, MS, MHA
Amba Coltman, BCSW, LICSW
Pamela Duchene, DNSc, RN
Nancy A. Dineen, RN, MSN
Marybeth Duffy, MSW, LICSW
Anna C. Foster, RN, BSW
Janice L. Gibeau, RN, Ph.D., CS
Phebe Goldman, RN, BSN, MPH
Jack Haynes, MSW, LICSW
Kathleen Kinneen, MSW, MBA, LICSW
Barbara Kotz, MSW, LICSW
Kathy MacDonald, LICSW
Joyce Marshall, RN
Noreen G. Mattis, RN, M.Ed.
Jane B. Mayer, MSW, LICSW
Susan A. Myers, MSW, LICSW
Caralyn Nash, LICSW
Kathleen M. Orr, MSW, CCM
Patricia Palermo, MS, RN
Ellen Parker, MSW
Elizabeth Reilinger, Ph.D.
Jean Robbins, LICSW, CDP
Joyce MacDonald Shannon, RN, MS
Irene Sommers, BSN, MBA
Linda A. Souza, BSN
Sheila Upchurch, MSW
Gail Kuhn Weissman, RN, Ed.D., FAAN
Susan Lacey Williams, RN, MSW, LICSW

All of the above-named individuals honed our minds for this book. Our spirits were tended to by others. To David, Stu, and Sandy we owe those precious gifts of patience, space, good humor, and the willingness to adjust their lives to our work. To our children, John, Andy, Glen,

Marshall, Christine, and Todd, we owe support and a constant, quiet cheering section. We thank our friends for their unfailing support and their gentle questioning of our ideas, coupled with an exuberant belief in our abilities, both as individuals and as a team.

J. W. H.
C. W. P.
N. W. V.

Contributors

Valerie A. Hamel, MS, RNC
Women's Health Care Nurse Practitioner
Women's Medical Center
Cranston, RI

Carol J. McMahon Morin, RN, MS, CS
Family Nurse Practitioner in
   private collaborative practice
Newburyport, MA

Ellen Trabka, RN, MS, CS
Family Nurse Practitioner
Santa Fe, NM

Susan L. Williams, RN, MSW, LICSW
Supervisor of Community Social Work Services
VNA Health Services
Franklin Medical Center
Greenfield, MA

CHAPTER 1

Introduction: Managed Care Is Here to Stay

MANAGED CARE: AN OXYMORON FOR NURSES AND SOCIAL WORKERS?

Managed health care and behavioral health care have set the nursing and social work professions on their ears. Both professions are reeling from privatization, cutbacks in staff, the rationing of services to society's most needy and at-risk people, and a lack of respect for professional education and training that was formerly held in high repute. Not only has managed care caused insecurity within the nursing and social work professions, but it has fueled competition and turf animosity between the two professions.

The community is and will continue to be the most significant arena for health and behavioral health services delivery. In this arena, nurses and social workers must collaborate, coordinating their unique services into a seamless package, and communicate selflessly on behalf of the health and behavioral health client. Ironically, this is where and how nurses and social workers began in the early 20th century, collaborating almost interchangeably in the larger community. Both professions lost the collaborative knack, became bureaucratized in both settings and ideas, and became competitive as each sought higher status, which was frequently conferred by the medical profession.

This book proposes a model for nurse–social worker collaboration as caregivers and services deliverers in communities in the 21st century. We call the model the Biopsychosocial Individual and Systems Intervention Model (BISIM). In essence, the proposed model brings nursing and social work back together where they began—in the communities where people live their lives. That interventions designed and delivered in community settings over the life span have been found to be the most effective and efficient meets precisely the two most important mandates of managed care, which are effectiveness and efficiency. The proposed model, there-

1

fore, amply meets the requisites of managed care; engages the thrust for excellence in professional practice on the part of nursing and social work; and, most important of all, satisfies the consumer's need for accessible, affordable, relevant, and quality services delivered in their own communities.

MANAGED CARE: WHO MANAGES, WHO CARES?

Managed care has evolved over the last 20 years and is now fraught with controversy. The managed care concept has several unique features:

- Imposes limits on consumer choice of provider;
- Attempts to modify utilization patterns through coordination of service delivery;
- Shares risks with providers to alter provider behavior or to encourage new service formation;
- Shifts the incentive for structural changes and cost containment to the primary provider rather than leaving it to the individual consumer. (Hurley & Freund, 1988; cited in Raiff & Shore, 1993, p. 149)

The emphasis is on provider or payer-driven health and behavioral health care, thus removing almost all cost control and much treatment judgment from professionals actually delivering the services.

One of the major sources of conflict between managed care systems and the nursing and social work professions is that in managed care systems, the "managed" concept prevails, whereas in professions such as nursing and social work, the "care" concept is most important. Professions exist to provide services; managed health exists largely to provide profits. The issue is starkly drawn: Care for all as needed or the bottom line? The clash between two seemingly dichotomous cultures is audible and visible in both the professional literature and the popular press.

The professional literature is currently replete with hotly debated issues around the privatization of health and behavioral health services delivery; rationing of care; lack of access to care by the most at-risk and needy populations; questions about what is the role of so-called "alternative" therapies; partnerships, alliances, takeovers, and downsizing; ethics and value clashes about who should have access to readily available computerized information about clients; protocols, assessment tools, and proprietorship of these instruments; and outcome-measurement questions such as who decides who did what and how well, and are client satisfaction measures alone sufficient to calibrate outcomes?

Headlines in popular and professional presses also underline the conflicts on an almost daily basis:

- "Manage with Care"
- "NASW's Position on Managed Care: We Are Unequivocally 'Pro-Client' "
- "Report on Managed Care Cites Concerns"
- "Child Welfare: Under New Management?"
- "Seattle Officials Seeking to Establish a Subsidized Natural Medicine Clinic"
- "Health Maintenance Organizations Are Turning to Spiritual Healing"
- "Mental Health: Does Therapy Help?"
- "Managing Managed Care"
- "HMOs May Not Always Be Best for Long-Term Ills"
- "Mental Health Providers Confront the Future"
- "Employers' Health Costs Are Stabilizing"
- "Hospitals Court Foreign Patients to Fill Beds"
- "Behavioral Health Involvement High"
- "Failing Health"

NURSING AND SOCIAL WORK UNITE TO LEAD IN MANAGED CARE SYSTEMS

Nursing and social work must put all of this together and work out a viable collaboration that both manages and cares for the community. Balancing the concrete and the conceptually complex is the task of each of these professions singly and in collaboration. This book provides a model for this collaboration.

The model assumes that the nurse–social worker will be both managing and caring. The model factors out, within an advanced case management framework, which of the two professions takes responsibility for which specific aspects of a case. The model also indicates where task performance may be performed jointly or equally by either profession.

Although nursing and social work share a common historic development, their professional alliance in the community is not now, as it was at the beginning of this century, logical and easy. Managed care is predicated on competition, particularly among providers, such as nursing and social work, for restricted services funding. Social workers perceive that nurses have taken over all of the important roles in managed care, such as team leader and case manager. Nurses feel that they are educated as well, or better, than social workers along the entire biopsychosocial intervention continuum (the "bio" part is uncontested as belonging to nursing; it is the "psychosocial" area where social workers feel most encroached on by nursing). Both professions, therefore, accuse the other of taking over and poaching on contested turf. It is to managed care's advantage to let this marketplace competition sort out the most effective services (frequently seen as the most extensive services contained in one package) for the lowest price, in essence, getting the biggest bang for the buck.

It is up to nursing and social work to unite in the community to show managed care systems that a nurse–social work collaborative team is both the most effective and most efficient way to deliver quality services to at-risk populations in the community. This book describes and analyzes a model for implementing this collaborative effort.

OUTLINE OF THE BOOK

Chapter 2 expands on this brief discussion of one part of the revolution in American health care—managed care. Chapter 3 returns to the historic roots of nursing and social work, roots from the same community tree that produced the branches for the many varieties of nursing and social work practice. Chapter 4 describes findings from the survey of chief nurses and social workers conducted in a range of health and behavioral health settings, which formed the basis for the BISIM, which is overviewed in chapter 5. Chapter 6 operationalizes the BISIM and gives case examples of how nurses and social workers can collaborate in the community. Chapter 7 questions the viability of traditional assessment and diagnostic models for current and future community health and behavioral health practice.

Chapter 8 takes a fond look back at the view from the hospital, where so many of us in health services learned at least part of our trade. Chapter 9 then brings us back into the community, where we propose to carry out the BISIM. Chapter 10 takes a look at new roles for the physician in the collaborative community health services delivery system we propose. In chapter 11, we look ahead to education-and-training needs as well as research imperatives for nurses and social workers in the next century. Finally, we look at some of the ethical concerns that will need constant vigilance in this new model of nurse–social worker collaboration in the community.

REFERENCES

Hurley, R. E., & Freund, D. A. (1988). A typology of Medicaid managed care. *Medical Care, 26,* 764–774.

Raiff, N. R., & Shore, B. K. (1993). *Advanced case management. New strategies for the nineties.* Newbury Park, CA: Sage.

CHAPTER 2

Revolution and Chaos in American Health Care

Health care in the United States has been under siege and is undergoing a revolution. The entire picture of health care delivery has changed dramatically. Health care has experienced significant changes and will continue to change as the war to gain control of the cost of health care continues. However, with change comes opportunity.

Health care has become very expensive and consumes more of the gross national product (GNP) than is considered healthy for the economic well-being of the country. We spend more per capita on health care than any other nation. Industry and government, which actually bear most of the cost of health care through health insurance for employees, are forcing change. Managed care systems are seen as an important mechanism to hold down health care costs.

Control of medical care itself seems to have shifted from physicians and hospitals to third-party payers and managed care organizations. Business and finance today dictate health care practices. As much health care as possible has shifted from the hospital to the community. These changes have helped to bring escalating costs under control.

Only the acutely ill are now in hospitals. All others are cared for either in a subacute or long-term facility or at home. For subacute and long-term care and for community-based agencies, this has been an opportunity for growth and recognition of their importance; subacute and long-term care facilities are full and expanding. These facilities maximize use of trained workers and are able to hire few professionals. Is this a real cost savings or another example of cost shifting?

For the chronically ill or persons unable to care for themselves, care in a long-term facility, subacute facility, or at home may be the best way to receive care. To die at home with hospice care can be more humane than dying in a hospital or long-term care facility and is preferred by many people. To take home a small, but healthy premature baby is possible and may be best for both the infant and the family. To have cataract surgery and go home within hours saves the patient from staying overnight in a strange and often frightening environment. The person with schizophrenia is able to live at home after a brief initial acute hospitalization and is very comfortable there.

But the question that needs to be raised more often is whether these changes occur at personal cost to all of us? What has happened to the people involved, the patients, their families, and the caregivers? Who makes these decisions? Do patients and families really have the choice? Who is responsible for caring for those with long-term illnesses? Can persons who are dying stay in a care facility if they wish? Or if their families or significant others wish? Can a preterm infant stay in the hospital if the mother is incapable of caring for such a young infant or if the home is a rat-infested, unheated tenement? Who gives the eye drops and cares for persons after cataract surgery who are scared, cannot get the eye drops in, and have no one to help them? Must the family care for the mentally ill member who totally disrupts their lives? These are questions about choice. They are also questions about saving money and about opportunity.

Families, significant others, neighbors, and friends are called on to administer care once given in hospitals. They may willingly welcome the opportunity to care for a loved one, or they may not. This is a shifting of burden of care and cost. Lost work days, lost vacation days, or lost jobs are expensive to the individual's and the nation's economy, but not to the health care system. Giving care for an extended time at home can be extremely difficult and lead to loss of personal choices and stress for those who are assuming the burden of care. What happens to those needing care at home who have no one to help them? What about those family members who need relief for continual caregiving? Community agencies and private businesses have an unprecedented opportunity to provide the care and fill the gaps that exist in health care.

Professionals within hospitals are being asked to be responsible for the care of acutely ill patients with a mix of a minimum of professional persons and maximum of unlicensed and minimally trained persons, both in social work and nursing. Professional career opportunities are diminishing in acute care; salaries and benefits are remaining at the same level or shrinking. Those who remain in acute care will be called on increasingly to manage other workers instead of administering hands-on care.

Leisure time is lost because the salaried professional is expected to work harder and longer. Large health care organizations are providing on-site services such as car washing, laundry, dry cleaning, convenience stores, and so on. Do employers care about their employees and are therefore trying to make life easier for them, or do these conveniences mean they want their employees to have less need to go home early or have time off because they can take care of their chores on breaks from work?

Consistently larger work loads and uncertainty concerning the future are stressful. Will this stress lead to increased illness among the formerly well? Will new illnesses arise? What are the choices available and what decisions must these professionals make? Where are the opportunities today? New business and professional opportunities are there for those who are creative and motivated to seize the opportunities in subacute, long-term, and community-based care. Further education, training, or both will enable health care professionals to assume new roles. Entrepreneurial professionals will help fill the gaps that exist in health care today.

Social work is making the shift to the community more rapidly than nursing. The opportunities are there for both nursing and social work professionals, and if they combine their energy and creativity, they can gain a foothold in controlling and creating models for health care in the community.

MANAGED CARE

Owens stated, "Managed health care is an entity that seeks to control the cost of health care by using a select group of providers, who have agreed to a predetermined payment, with the clinical intervention being managed via utilization and/or a case management process" (1996, p. 1). Similarly, Vogel (1993) defined managed care as a "means of providing healthcare services within a defined network of healthcare providers who are given the responsibility to manage and provide quality, cost-effective health-care" (p. 4). The goal of managed care is not merely to lower costs, but to ensure that subscribers receive maximum value from the planning and delivery of health care (Hicks, Stallmeyer, & Coleman, 1993, p. 1). The financial basis for managed care is prospective financing (Schultz, 1991, p. 16).

Managed care organizations vary widely and include, but are not limited to, health maintenance organizations (HMOs), preferred provider organizations (PPOs), employer-negotiated arrangements, government-sponsored organizations, physician-hospital organizations (Welge, 1992, p. 23; Owens, 1996, pp. 7–17, 31–39), and health care systems. These managed care providers aim to negotiate the best contracts with individuals and businesses handling heath care coverage, physicians, hospitals, therapists, pharmacists, and other service or product vendors. Managed care wants profits without creating barriers to quality health care and must stay within federal, state, and local regulations and other legal constraints (Welge, 1992, p. 24).

HISTORIC ROOTS OF MANAGED CARE

The concept of managed care is not new. As early as the 13th and 16th centuries, organizations mutualized costs and delivered health care to certain trade professions (Drew, 1990, p. 145). The Mayo Clinic, begun in 1887, grew into the first large group practice (Hawkins & Higgins, 1993, p. 128).

The Ross–Loos Clinic in Los Angeles and the Elk City Farmers Cooperative Association in Elk City, Oklahoma are credited with the formal founding of managed care in 1929 (Falkson, 1980, p. 17). The Ross–Loos Plan contracted with the city of Los Angeles to provide prepaid health care for the city's water workers (Falkson, 1980, p. 17; MacColl, 1966, pp. 11–12). The Elk City Cooperative, a consumer-controlled health plan whose members were farmers, fought for 20 years with county and state medical societies who tried to obstruct their progress (Falkson, 1980, p. 17; MacColl, 1966, pp. 20–23). In California in the 1930s, Kaiser was established as a leader in managed care on the west coast, and in the 1940s the Health Insurance Plan of New York brought managed care east (Falkson, 1980, pp. 18–19).

Government involvement in health care was limited. In 1965 the government began to play a large role in health care with the passage of Titles XVIII and XIX of the Social Security Act, part of President Johnson's Great Society program. It was designed as an antipoverty program (Oot-Giromini, Morris, & Feather, 1990, p. 415), but the consequence was a tremendous increase in medical service utilization and cost. The explosion of new products and pharmaceuticals, along with a hospital building boom, sent health care costs skyrocketing (Ennis & Meneses, 1996, p. 55). The public viewed health care as free. Employers paid for health insurance for their employees, and the government paid for the elderly and the poor (Owens, 1996, p. 2).

Ways were sought to cut high health care delivery costs due to the cost of the fee-for-service payment method. During the Nixon administration, managed care was endorsed and promoted under the Part C addition to Titles XVIII and XIX of the Social Security Act and other legislation (Falkson, 1980, p. 37). Pub. L. No. 93-222 was passed in Congress in 1973 authorizing the use of federal funds (loans and grants) to aid in the development of HMOs (Hicks, et al., 1993, p. 9). Other provisions of the law included the requirement that HMOs provide comprehensive services and additional optional choices. Open enrollments were mandated, as was use of community ratings[1] to set premiums. Employers were required to offer an HMO option if available (Hicks, et al., 1993, p. 9). Since then, the community rating system and optional services are no longer necessary (Langwell, 1990, p. 74).

Reform was slow as medical societies lobbied, the public demanded choices for both provider and access, and per-member (capitation) rates were difficult to establish (Ennis & Meneses, 1996, p. 55). The Tax Equity and Fiscal Responsibility Act of 1982 enabled Medicare patients to enroll in HMOs; consequently over 1.2 million Medicare recipients have enrolled in managed care systems (Ennis & Meneses, 1996, p. 55).

The first PPOs, like HMOs, began in the early 1900s. In Washington and Oregon, an insurance company negotiated preferred rates for subscribers through worker compensation. Outpatient and inpatient services by physicians and other providers were included. In the 1930s, California Physicians Services contracted to purchaser groups. Finally, in the 1970s, the PPO structure was initiated in California by the Foundation for Medical Care Plan and marketed to employer groups. PPOs, like HMOs, have grown in the 1980s and 1990s. It is controversial whether this alternative will continue to meet cost controls (Owens, 1996, p. 32).

Managed care has survived due to many factors. Health care costs directly affect industry and government (tax payer), who pay the bills for employee benefits. The public has demanded health-care reform. Large numbers of HMOs have converted from nonprofit to for profit (Langwell, 1990, p. 73). By the year 2000, it is projected that 70% of the population will be enrolled in some form of managed care, but the HMOs themselves will shrink in number through consolidation (Ennis & Meneses, 1996, p. 55).

Managed care has controlled costs mainly through shorter hospital stays, admission testing, second opinions, same-day surgery, discharge planning, and utilization review. Today and in the future, cost containment for outpatient services (Leyland, 1991, p. 165) is an additional focus. It includes referral authorization, provider incentives, provider networks, and drug formularies (Ennis & Meneses, 1996, p. 55).

Taylor and Kagay (1986) believe the membership of HMOs will continue to grow very rapidly as the HMOs are better able to satisfy the needs of the fee-for-service consumer; garner increasing employer support; incure decreasing physician hostility; and offer the increasing attrac-

---

[1]Community rating is an insurance term referring to actuarial risks in a community in which illnesses are averaged. High- and low-risk groups each receive the same risk rating, therefore, equal premiums are set (Falkson, 1980, p. 128).

tiveness of prepaid insurance in an era of increasing insurance cost, copayments, and deductibles. PPOs will remain strong and competitive due to the combination of prepayment and traditional system features. There will be more competition from ambulatory care services, urgent care centers, and surgicenters (p. 88). Ennis and Meneses (1996) do not entirely agree and predict that increasingly people will use the more tightly controlled HMOs instead of the more loosely organized PPOs (p. 55).

TYPES OF MANAGED CARE

INDEMNITY INSURANCE PLANS

It has become increasingly difficult to distinguish among managed care choices. Traditional indemnity insurance plans do not include managed care; however, today almost all traditional indemnity health insurance plans have incorporated managing the health care services of their subscribers and utilization management techniques of managed care into their plans (Hicks, et al., 1993, p. 13). Traditional indemnity plans have two types of coverage, preestablished *cash payment* for services and *cost of services* utilized. Cash payment plans pay for services up to an established amount. There is no incentive to shop for services. With cost of services, the subscriber locates the provider from a selected list of providers and sites; only certain services are covered. It is not comprehensive insurance. This has led to overusage at locations that are covered (Hicks et al., 1993, pp. 5–6).

HEALTH MAINTENANCE ORGANIZATIONS

An HMO can be defined as a "comprehensive health care financing and delivery organization which provides or arranges for provision of covered health care services to a specified group of enrollees, at a fixed periodic payment through a panel or providers" (Massachusetts Nurses Association, 1995, p. 14). HMOs give their providers incentives to deliver health care efficiently. The financial incentives may include risking their personal salary or the group's salary if costs are too high, sharing the profits, and bonuses. Nonfinancial incentives are education concerning efficient use of resources, individualized feedback, participating in the planning, and administrative constraints (Hillman, 1989, pp. 85, 88, 91). HMOs operated at lower costs initially, primarily due to lower hospitalization utilization rates (Luft, 1978, pp. 1337, 1342; Taylor & Kagay, 1986, p. 84), but by the late 1980s some had losses (Gruber, Shadle, & Polich, 1988, p. 206).

An HMO's rate of increasing the cost to consumers is somewhat less than the rate of indemnity plans (Gruber et al., 1988, p. 207). However, the rate of cost-inflation growth in HMOs is the same rate as traditional insurance (Hillman, 1989, p. 84).

In general, HMOs have voluntary enrollment of members and are an organized system of health care in a given geographic location. The system includes physicians, hospitals services, and other health care providers. Subscriber payment is predetermined and paid by the employers who insure their workers or by the individual member (Owens, 1996, pp. 7–8). Subscriber copayments for visits to health care providers and pharmaceuticals are common. The HMO must meet federal or state requirements for minimum basic comprehensive health services (Owens, 1996, pp. 7–8).

HMOs may be licensed by the state or federal government. The minimum required benefits for federally licensed programs include a much broader range of services than do state licensed programs (Owens, 1996, p. 9). There are five basic types or models of licensed HMOs: staff, group, network, independent practice arrangement, and point of service. In the *staff model*, physicians are salaried employees of the HMO and they provide services in ambulatory care at the plan's center or centers (Owens, 1996, p. 10). In the *group model*, a group of physicians or multispecialty physicians contract to provide service through the HMO plan. These physicians may or may not also provide care outside the plan (Owens, 1996, pp. 10–11). In the *network model* the group model is expanded; the contracts are with one or more groups of physicians. The physician groups may be primary care physicians such as family practitioners, general practitioners, or internists; multispeciality groups; or both (Owens, 1996, p. 11). In the *independent practice arrangement*, physicians contract with small specialty groups and those in solo practice to provide services to its HMO members. The physicians may see members and nonmembers (Owens, 1996, p. 12). In the *point of service* arrangement, HMO members may receive services outside the network, but must pay a high copayment or deductible (Owens, 1996, p. 12). Many HMOs are hybrids. An example is an independent practice arrangement based in Birmingham, Alabama called Complete Health, which contracts with 47 hospitals and 2,316 HMO physician providers to provide services throughout the state. This is joint venture between the University of Alabama and a group of business leaders begun in 1986 (Widra & Fottler, 1992, p. 206).

There are also nonlicensed systems models that have adopted some of the management and control systems of HMOs such as group practice with walls, physician–hospital organization, managed services organization, and specialty health maintenance organizations. Lastly, there are integrated delivery and integrated network systems. *Group practice with-*

out walls is an arrangement created for administration and management cost sharing for individual physician practices. The individual physicians contract with the HMO and are autonomous (Owens, 1996, p. 13). The *physician–hospital organization* integrates hospital and physician services and management. This legal arrangement between the hospital and physician works toward cost containment and facilitates contracting with HMOs (Owens, 1996, p. 14). A *managed services organization* is an administrative entity that manages many of the services that are typically part of managed care such as contracting, case management, utilization management, and information systems. The managed services organization is comprised of individual physicians, physician groups, independent practice arrangements, hospitals, and physician-hospital organizations (Owens, 1996, pp. 14–15). The *specialty health maintenance organization model* is not really an HMO at all. This HMO is created to provide specialty care only such as dentistry or mental health. These specialties were not included in the original legislation (Owens, 1996, pp. 15–16).

PREFERRED PROVIDER ORGANIZATION

''A preferred provider organization is best defined as a plan that contracts with independent providers at a discount for services'' (Owens, 1996, p. 31). Subscribers are given financial incentives to choose care from a special group of providers but are not limited in their ability to choose when and from whom services are provided (Hicks et al., 1993, p. 12). This type of plan is something of a hybrid between HMOs and standard indemnity insurance plans (Hicks et al., 1993, p. 3).

The PPO may be insurance sponsored, a physician–hospital organization, third-party administrator, or employer sponsored. In the *insurance-sponsored* PPO, an insurance company creates its own benefit or product. The insurance company may choose to develop, purchase, or rent a network of providers and markets that network to the subscribers. Examples are Cigna and Met Life Healthplans (Owens, 1996, pp. 33–34). The *physician–hospital organization* PPO is a formalized network that manages the hospital–physician relationship. It is a collaboration between physicians. The hospital provides a network of services, and the physician oversees claims and utilization review and is a participant in the policy and procedure formulation. Examples are Sutter and Humana Health Care Systems of California (Owens, 1996, p. 34). Another PPO is the *third-party administrator*. A third-party administrator is a company created by entrepreneurs, other companies, or trust funds to provide services for administrative duties, claims processing, and case management. Beech Street in California and Value Health in Washington are examples. An *employer-sponsored*

PPO creates its own health plan and develops its own network of providers. This PPO may develop a relationship with others PPOs or contract with traditional payers. Honeywell and Xerox Corporations and Southern California Edison Company use this structure (Owens, 1996, p. 34).

EXCLUSIVE PROVIDER ORGANIZATIONS

Exclusive provider organizations combine characteristics of both the HMO and the PPO and are basically indemnity plans. The prepaid primary care physician gatekeeps services, but subscribers can access other providers in the network without a referral. If the subscriber goes outside the network for health care, the subscriber pays a higher copayment or deductible (Owens, 1996, pp. 37–38).

EMPLOYER NEGOTIATED ARRANGEMENTS

Some employers find they can cut costs by using self-insured in-house health plans. They use the same techniques for cost cutting as HMOs and may employ an HMO management company to administer the plan (Ellwood, 1988, p. 88). Employers are also encouraging their employees to choose the lowest cost health insurance plans by contributing only what the lowest priced HMO costs. The employer negotiates the best price with the HMO (Tweed, 1994, p. 27).

GOVERNMENT-SPONSORED ORGANIZATIONS

The U.S. government may be the single largest payer of health care costs. Medicare purchases health care for the elderly and the Medicaid (matching state and federal funds) program purchases care for the poor (Owens, 1996, p. 19). Increasingly, both these programs are being handled through contracts with HMOs or other managed care organizations instead of fee for service.

HEALTH CARE SYSTEMS

A health care system, a consolidation of hospitals, physicians, insurance companies, medical supply companies, and others for cost effective health care delivery (and the hopeful survival of its members), continues to be a growing trend. Large integrated national medical firms (such as Columbia HCA Healthcare Corporation) integrate services both vertically and horizontally. Vertical integration may include an insurance company, physicians, medical supply businesses, a hospital, and more. Horizontal integration is when one hospital integrates with other hospital(s) and whatever is integrated with it (Ellwood, 1988, p. 87).

CASE MANAGEMENT

Managed health care organizations utilize care management as a mechanism for improving the quality of care, reducing inappropriate use of services, and controlling costs (Hicks et al., 1993, p. 49). Client populations have varied greatly according to age, relative health status, and sociodemographic characteristics. In particular, case managers handle members with catastrophic injury and illness, those with disabling or chronic conditions, and high-risk high-use members (Like, 1988, p. 175). Those who will cost the managed care plan a large amount of money per year or who are likely to exceed life benefits are also included in case management (Hicks et al., 1993, p. 49).

Case management is a client and provider relationship in which the provider coordinates, advocates, and integrates services for individuals, families, and groups (Bower, 1992, p. 3; Schultz, 1991, p. 16). The goal is to make health care more holistic and less fragmented, particularly for patients with complex health care needs (Schultz, 1991, p. 16). It includes alternatives to inpatient care services such as at home professional nursing care, healthcare, homemaker services, speech therapy, nutritional counseling, hospice care, and extended care facilities (Boland, 1993, p. 190). Regardless of the exact type of case management, all case managers coordinate health care (Bower, 1992, p. 3).

Case management is not new. It has been used in public health nursing, social service agencies, rehabilitation settings, and by insurance companies for decades (Zander, 1990, p. 199). The setting and context for case management varies more widely today, including the former settings plus nursing practice, independent practice, community agencies, maternal-child and mental health settings (Bower, 1992, p. 4), HMOs, PPOs, and hospitals. The case management arrangement may be employer based, insurance based, or part of workers' compensation programs (Bower, 1992, p. 4).

Crawley and Till studied case management and found that with case management in a 540-bed teaching hospital there was improved quality of care, increased patient and staff satisfaction, and decreased costs and lengths of stay (1995, pp. 116–119).

HOSPITAL CASE MANAGEMENT

Case management within hospitals includes short-term components, long-term components, or both. Short-term case management aids in the transition from the hospital; long-term assists for an extended period. Hospital-based case management generally emphasizes resource control, whereas community-based case management stresses client advocacy in finding scarce resources (Williams, Warrick, Christianson, & Netting, 1994, p. 131). Critical pathways predict the key incidents that must occur, the expected time frame, and the appropriate length of stay. Progress is measured at regular intervals (perhaps as often as every 8 hours), and adjustments made as needed. Cost and length of stay are measurable outcomes of case management (Bower, 1992, pp. 43–44).

Both social work and nursing are needed for this work. The social worker has the background necessary to coordinate and broker community services. The nurse carries out the assessment and care planning (Williams, et al., 1994, p. 137). Case management ideally begins before hospitalization (Lamprey & Corcoran, 1991, p. 412). Utilization management (instead of utilization review) begins in the preadmission period, continues during an admission, and includes follow-up after discharge (Lamprey & Corcoran, 1991, pp. 412–413).

COMMUNITY CASE MANAGEMENT

Case management in the community follows the public health model. Health departments use case management to identify, evaluate, diagnose, and treat those in need of services (Bower, 1992, pp. 41–42). Case management is also utilized at nursing centers or other health care centers within the community (Bower, 1992, pp. 30, 38). Case management serves as an entry point into the health care system for comprehensive health care (Bower, 1992, pp. 41–42); case managers make home visits and provide a variety of services (Bower, 1992, p. 38). They establish long-term relationships with patients and may work with them across settings during and between exacerbations (Bower, 1992, p. 30). Often children, pregnant women, those with chronic illnesses, and elderly persons are the focus of this type of case management (Bower, 1992, pp. 37–40, 41–42). Again, both nursing and social work are needed. The unique focus and contribution of each, plus their united strength, provide the best and most comprehensive care.

WHO ARE THE CASE MANAGERS?

Physicians As Case Managers

Within managed care, physicians are case managers (Like, 1988, p. 174); their role is often perceived as that of gatekeepers (Boland, 1993, p. 156;

Somers, 1983, p. 301). Physician case managers serve as the patient's primary physician; referrals for specialist services are made by the primary physician. This is a condition imposed by third-party payers and works best in a capitated system (Somers, 1983, pp. 301–302). Like (1988) proposed that case management by physicians go beyond primary care management, and that if physicians work closely with other social and human services, they can improve the services to include psychosocial, contextual, and biomedical aspects of care (pp. 174, 177).

Primary care physicians act as primary care case managers for Medicaid clients. Only services authorized by the primary physician are reimbursed, except in the event of a true emergency. Only three states do not require Medicaid recipients to choose a primary care case manager. Some states pay physicians a small monthly fee called a case management fee for being case managers. Clients may choose their own primary or physician sponsors (Fox & Neuschler, 1993, pp. 563–565).

Nurses As Case Managers

Bower stated: "Case management has emerged as a strategy to focus on the problems and needs of clients, as well as the families and friends who support their problems and needs, while maintaining a balance between outcome, cost, and process. The overall purpose of case management is to advocate for the patient through coordination of care, which reduces fragmentation and ultimately cost" (1992, p. 2). Historically, nurses have been case managers in psychiatric and public health settings and when insurance companies wanted to control costs they hired nurses as case managers. Today, the nurse as case manager is employed in many contexts and settings (Bower, 1992, pp. 2–3).

In comparison to the physician as case manager, the nurse's scope is broader. It includes intake and assessment, care-plan development and implementation, referral and follow up, coordination of cases, further assessment, planning termination, reporting and recording, worker supervision, and quality assurance (Shipske, 1987, p. 4). The nurse case manager in most settings carries out the following roles: liaison, facilitator, negotiator, educator, monitor, reporter, evaluator of outcomes, gatekeeper (Bower, 1992, pp. 5, 21–22), patient advocate, caregiver, coordinator, and broker (Davis, 1996, p. 193). Bower (1992) described case management as a role, a system, a service, a technology, and a process (pp. 4–5).

Zander (1990) believes nurses are better than physicians as case managers because they are generalists, detail oriented, and are excellent care managers. They have formal training in all aspects of health care (p. 201) and are able to draw on their educational backgrounds.

Social Workers As Case Managers

"Social work case management is a method of providing services whereby a professional social worker assesses the needs of the client and the client's family, when appropriate, and arranges, coordinates, monitors, evaluates, and advocates for a package of multiple services to meet the specific client's complex needs" (National Association of Social Workers [NASW], 1992, p. 5). Social work case management is linked historically to social casework in which the social worker works with the client directly, and family indirectly, in meeting social service needs; the focus is both on the person and the environment. Today social work case management also encompasses efficient and cost-effective methods for delivery of multiple service to target populations (NASW, 1992, p. 4). The focus is bringing services to the most difficult and vulnerable populations (Raiff & Shore, 1993, p. 15). Interventions are both micro and macro—they occur at both client and systems levels. The social worker develops and maintains a therapeutic relationship with a client with the goal of optimizing the client's functioning (NASW, 1992, p. 5).

The role of the social worker is complex and calls for a variety of skills such as outreach worker, evaluator, advocate, consultant, broker, diagnostician, planner, therapist, and community organizer (NASW, 1992, pp. 8, 12). Greene (1992) saw social worker case managers as those who identified clients and provided outreach, assessed and diagnosed individuals and families, identified resources and planned services, linked clients to needed services, implemented and coordinated services, monitored service delivery, advocated to obtain services, and evaluated services and service delivery (pp. 17–23). The social work case manager must understand the client population and practice setting (cultural, socioeconomic, gender, racial, and sexual orientation) that may affect use of services, the system of resources and interrelationships among them, and fiscal and other consequences of using services (NASW, 1992, p. 9).

FUTURE OF MANAGED CARE

Jennings and O'Leary predicted that the 1990s will be "the decade of integration" (1994, p. 39). As they pointed out, we tried cooperative planning in the 1970s without success; then in the 1980s the costly strategy of diversification was attempted for about 5 years (Jennings & O'Leary, 1994, p. 39). Today we have mergers, acquisitions, and consolidation of all facets of health care. This trend is likely to continue.

Organizations are being restructured as locally integrated delivery networks. Integrated delivery networks or systems utilize an integrated financing mechanism or capitation payment system. Capitation is payment based on enrollment, not the services. Providers must be willing to accept and manage financial risks. The focus is on wellness, prevention, and early intervention (Jennings & O'Leary, 1994, pp. 39–40). The purpose of the network is to manage health care services utilization from tertiary inpatient care to primary care and all related services. Information systems, utilization data, and financial management are shared. This type of system can be developed by an HMO, a hospital, physician group, or traditional insurer. The technically nonlegal entity links or integrates physicians, hospitals, other clinicians, support and administrative staff, and services (Owens, 1996, p. 16). The insurance company may or may not be a part of the network (Jennings & O'Leary, 1994, pp. 45–46).

Jennings and O'Leary (1994, pp. 40–41) stated that the collaborative strategies of the integrated delivery network include both vertical and horizontal integration. Vertical integration is the development of a continuum of care services. This ensures that the subscribers' full range of health care needs are met by the network. The array of services includes prevention; screening; education; specialized and primary ambulatory care; acute, subacute, and long-term inpatient care; and home health care. Physicians and hospitals must collaborate for this to happen.

Horizontal integration is actually collaboration, which we all recognize as mergers, acquisitions, and consolidation. Care must be taken that competition is not diminished through these collaborations, and that they are not in violation of antitrust laws (Jennings & O'Leary, 1994, p. 43). Horizontal integration may take the form of an alliance, managed care company, or holding company. In the alliance model, no organization relinquishes control over its governance, assets, and management to participate; the alliance is jointly owned and controlled by the members. The managed care company is jointly owned and controlled by the sponsoring independent organizations. The goal is mutual benefit to all sponsors, but the sponsor may find the managed care company dictates policy to them. When a holding company is the model, a parent company holds control over subsidiary corporations. All individual assets, governance, and management are relinquished (Jennings & O'Leary, 1994, pp. 43–45).

Shapleigh (1993, pp. 27–28) advocated a closed-loop approach to hospital contracting with managed care. As hospitals negotiate contracts, they must have sophisticated information systems that provide them with strategic, financial, and patient care information. The health care agency must know its true costs, whether its rate structure covers the cost, and its net and gross margins. The exact cost for an obstetric or coronary bypass patient should be readily available. An agency must be able to set a price to take to the bargaining table. When contracting with managed care, the care agency must clearly define what services it is expected to provide, its obligations when subscribers need transfer to another facility, the utilization review process, quality assurance expectations, liability risks for a mistaken utilization review decision, mechanisms of claim processing, renewal terms, and termination procedures (Rosenbloom, 1995, pp. 30–31).

CLOSING THOUGHTS

Shindul-Rothschild, in an article concerning the economics of managed care, concluded, "the compelling evidence we have so far is an undisputed conclusion that it doesn't save money and there are serious problems with access and quality of care" (1995, p. 6). The premium cost to customers is less in managed care arrangements. The lower cost is not due to greater efficiency. In fact, the administrative costs are approximately 13% higher than fee-for-service arrangements. The savings are from providing less health care, particularly to women and children. Society must make sure that the weakest and most disadvantaged among us receive health care; currently we are locking them out of the system because of their inability to pay (Shindul-Rothschild, 1995, pp. 4, 6).

Caregivers are torn between autonomy when giving care to their patients and compromise with the managed care company paying the bill. The provider is clearly liable, and case reviewers may not be totally familiar with the nuances of the care needed. Discount medicine invites ultimately higher costs. Patients need nurses and social workers to be their advocates in the managed care systems (Weingart, 1991, pp. 40–41). Is managed care giving the best care possible or giving cut-rate care?

Weingart (1991) proposed that social workers and nurses can only act as true advocates if they document daily why the particular setting is the choice for the patient who is being treated, why the specific treatment modalities are being used, and why continuing the treatment is necessary. Documented treatment plans must include short- and long-term goals with time frames (critical pathways). They must be familiar with research concerning outcomes for similar conditions. A staff member should accompany reviewers during patient interviews and chart reviews. Reviewers should give notice ahead of time and records should be kept of the reviewers' activities. Reviews should not interfere with health care delivery. Information should be restricted to objective data and not released without proper authorization. Decisions to refuse needed treatment should be contested, and patients should seek legal counsel if the appeal is denied. Unresolved grievances must be reported to the state insurance commission.

There is concern that clinical research is one of the hidden casualties of managed-care-for-profit health care. Managed care is directly or indirectly denying researchers across the country money and access to patients. Clinical studies are necessary to understand diseases and to perfect drugs, treatments, and therapies. Managed care is eliminating research to reduce costs and, at worst case, its patients are not allowed to participate in clinical trials unless total care is paid for. Managed care is reluctant to share knowledge that could benefit all caregivers because of the desire for a competitive edge over others. Maybe for-profit managed care should be banned altogether (Gordon, 1996, pp. D1–D2).

No one knows the future, but controversy will remain concerning managed care. What does seem clear is that in the immediate future, more people will be cared for by some form of managed care. It does not seem likely that national health insurance is going to happen any time soon. We need to find a middle ground, somewhere between managed care and its incentive to undertreat and fee-for-service care with its incentive to overtreat (Wood, 1995, p. 15). As Federa and Camp (1994) stated,

> Managed care has evolved in response to severe economic and sociodemo-graphic pressure. It seemingly has evolved haphazardly with a dizzying array of model and options. Understandably, it did so to address the disparate characteristics of provider and consumer markets. Managed care may continue to show growing pains in novice markets and perhaps restructuring in sophisticated markets. What is clear is that the nation is primed for a certain degree of change, and that managed care, in its multiple forms, is likely to be the direction it takes. (p. 7)

Health care providers cannot allow the quality of care to suffer as we all believe it has, as payers have increasingly fragmented professional care delivery and parceled out the fragments to the cheapest employee. Downskilling and downgrading health care is not fair to patients who are unable to evaluate the quality of the care themselves. Providers cannot allow profiteering in the health care industry. Large amounts of health care dollars pay for administration, marketing, and consultants, but this is the business of caring for human beings, not auto repair (Costello, 1994, p. 6). Nurses and social workers need to be truly patient centered and become partners with patients in planning health care to meet their individual needs.

History gives us a context in which to view the present and the future of health care in general and managed health care specifically. Nursing and social work together have long been a model of cooperation in the community setting. As we examine the present and look toward the future, it only seems fitting that we learn from the lessons from the past.

REFERENCES

Boland, P. (1993). Evolving managed care organizations and product innovation. In P. Boland (Ed.), *Making managed healthcare work* (pp. 151–192). Gaithersburg, MD: Aspen.

Bower, K. A. (1992). *Case management by nurses*. Washington, DC: American Nurses Publishing.

Costello, K. (1994). Managed competition vs. single payer: What's best for patients and RNs? *California Nurse, 90*(6), 6.

Crawley, W. D., & Till, A. H. (1995). Case management: More population-based data. *Clinical Nurse Specialist, 9*, 116–120.

Davis, V. (1996). Staff development for nurse case management. In E. L. Cohen (Ed.), *Nurse case management in the 21st century* (pp. 189–208). St. Louis, MO: Mosby.

Drew, J. C. (1990). Health maintenance organization: History, evolution, and survival. *Nursing and Health Care, 11*, 144–149.

Ellwood, P. M. (1988, January). Trends: Less and more integration, bundled services, rethinking IPAs. *Consultant,* pp. 86–95.

Ennis, W. J., & Meneses, P. (1996). Strategic planning for the wound care clinic in a managed care environment. *Ostomy/Wound Management, 42*(3), 54–62.

Falkson, J. (1980). *HMOs and the politics of the health system reform*. Chicago: American Hospital Association.

Federa, R. D., & Camp, T. L. (1994). The changing managed care market. *Journal of Ambulatory Medicine, 17*, 1–7.

Fox, P. D., & Neuschler, E. (1993). Managed care and Medicare and Medicaid. In P. Boland (Ed.), *Making managed healthcare work* (pp. 557–573). Gaithersburg, MD: Aspen.

Gordon, S. (1996, October 13). Is research being 'managed' out of existence. *Boston Globe,* pp. D1–D2.

Greene, R. R. (1992). Case management: An arena for social work practice. In B. S. Vourlekis & R. R. Greene (Eds.), *Social work case management* (pp. 11–25). New York: Aldine de Gruyter.

Gruber, L. R., Shadle, M., & Polich, C. L. (1988). From movement to industry: The growth of HMOs. *Health Affairs, 7*, 197–208.

Hawkins, J. W., & Higgins, L. P. (1993). *Nursing and the American health care delivery system*. New York: Tiresias.

Hicks, L. L., Stallmeyer, J. M., & Coleman, J. R. (1993). *Role of the nurse in managed care*. Washington, DC: American Nurses Publishing.

Hillman, A. L. (1989, July). What's known, what's not known. *Consultant,* pp. 84–85, 88, 91.

Jennings, M. C., & O'Leary, S. J. (1994). The role of managed care in integrated delivery networks. *Journal of Ambulatory Care Management, 17*(1), 39–47.

Lamprey, J., & Corcoran, C. K. (1991). Design and implementation of quality assurance. In P. Boland (Ed.), *Making managed healthcare work* (pp. 401–414). Gaithersburg, MD: Aspen.

Langwell, K. M. (1990). Structure and performance of health maintenance organizations: A review. *Health Care Financing Review, 12,* 71–79.

Leyland, A. (1991). Managed care in the 1990's. *Journal of Medical Practice Management, 6,* 161–165.

Like, R. C. (1988). Primary care case management: A family physician's perspective. *Quarterly Review Bulletin, 14*(6), 174–178.

Luft, H. S. (1978). How do health maintenance organizations achieve their savings? Rhetoric and evidence. *New England Journal of Medicine, 298*(24), 1336–1343.

MacColl, W. A. (1966). *Group practice and prepayment of medical care.* Washington, DC: Public Affairs Press.

Massachusetts Nurses Association. (1995, October/November). Glossary of managed care terms. *Massachusetts Nurse,* p. 14.

National Association of Social Workers. (1992). *National Association of Social Workers standards for social work case management* [Brochure]. Washington, DC: Author.

Oot-Giromini, B., Morris, E. J., & Feather, J. (1990). The economics of chronic wound care: An overview. In D. Kraser (Ed.), *Chronic wound care: A clinical source book for healthcare professionals* (pp. 415–422). King of Prussia, PA: Health Management Publications.

Owens, C. (1996). *Managed care organizations: Practical implications for medical practices and other providers.* New York: McGraw Hill Health Care Management.

Raiff, N. R., & Shore, B. K. (1993). *Advanced case management: New strategies for the nineties.* Newbury Park, CA: Sage.

Rosenbloom, A. (1995). Negotiating your managed care future. *Nursing Homes, 44*(3), 29–31.

Schultz, P. R. (1991). Managed care. *Washington Nurse, 21*(5), 16–17.

Shapleigh, C. (1993). An integrated approach to managed care contracting. *Health Care Financial Management, 47*(8), 27–30.

Shindul-Rothschild, J. (1995). The economics of managed care. *Massachusetts Nurse, 65*(9), 4, 6.

Shipske, G. (1987). An overview of case management supervision. *Caring, 6*(2), 4–7, 34–40, 42–44.

Somers, A. (1983). And who shall be the gatekeeper? The role of primary physician in the health care delivery system. *Inquiry, 20,* 301–313.

Taylor, H., & Kagay, M. (1986). The HMO report card: A closer look. *Health Affairs, 5*(1), 81–89.

Tweed, V. (1994, October). Making HMOs compete. *Business & Health,* pp. 27–38.

Vogel, D. E. (1993). *Family physicians and managed care: A view for the 90s.* Kansas City, MO: American Academy of Family Physicians Publication.

Weingart, M. (1991). Commercially managed healthcare: An experience. *Nursing Management, 22*(1), 40–41.

Welge, W. L. (1992). Managed care is limited by the information system. *Topics in Health Care Financing, 19*(2), 23–32.

Widra, L. S., & Fottler, M. D. (1992). Determinants of HMO success: The case of complete health. In M. Brown (Ed.), *Managed care: Strategies, networks, and management* (pp. 205–223). Gaithersburg, MD: Aspen.

Williams, F. G., Warrick, L. H., Christianson, J. B., & Netting, F. E. (1994). Critical factors for successful hospital-based case management. In M. Brown (Ed.), *Managed care: Strategies, networks, and management* (pp. 131–138). Gaithersburg, MD: Aspen Publishers.

Wood, C. T. (1995, September 5). Managed care is not health care. *Boston Globe*, p. 15.

Zander, K. (1990). Case management: A golden opportunity for whom? In J. C. McCloskey & H. K. Grace (Eds.), *Current issues in nursing* (pp. 199–204). St. Louis, MO: Mosby.

CHAPTER 3

The Settlement House Movement: A Historic Collaboration of Nurses and Social Workers

Social work and nursing evolved along a similar evolutionary path, intersecting often but never more obviously than in the settlement house movement of the late 19th and early 20th centuries in the United States. Members of these two professions were responsible for responding in a very direct and concrete manner to the chaos cities experienced because of urbanization, industrialization, and immigration. The collaboration exhibited by nurses and social workers was not confined to urban areas, however. Similar efforts were directed at the problems of poverty and disenfranchisement in rural areas. In this chapter we explore the evolution of collaboration between social work and nursing through the lens of the settlement house.

A COMMON LINEAGE

To pinpoint the beginning of social work and nursing on the timeline of human history is an elusive quest. The roots of both professions rest in the stirrings of compassion among early humans for the suffering and pain of their brothers and sisters. In social histories that have survived through oral traditions among societies that had no written history, human communities clearly cared for their members, and that caring included both the physical and psychosocial needs. The Civil War, often cited as a beginning point for the development of modern nursing, coincided with the publication of Florence Nightingale's *Notes on Nursing* (1860) and the dissemination of this volume in the United States, as well as the establishment of the first Nightingale training school for nurses in collaboration with St. Thomas' Hospital, London (Woodham-Smith, 1951). Clara

Barton, Dorothea Dix, Walt Whitman, Louisa May Alcott, and countless other less well known women (mostly) who served as volunteer nurses during the Civil War were as much social workers as they were nurses. Walt Whitman wrote of reading to soldiers and writing letters for them (1882/1971). Following the end of the war, Clara Barton (1912) spent several years helping families to locate the graves of their loved ones.

The charitable work that gave rise to the professions of social work and nursing was expressed in numerous settings including hospitals, orphanages, prisons, asylums for the mentally ill, and the community at large. Van Blarcom wrote of social workers being part of the team for maternity and infancy work under the Sheppard-Towner Act of 1921 (1929, pp. 416–417). Collaboration in the community occurred in rural and urban areas. With the development of the district nursing model of Great Britain, more commonly called public health nursing or visiting nursing in the United States, new opportunities for working together arose. Laura Gamble, Director of Nursing for the Cattaraugus County New York Board of Health and Josephine Brown, Associate Field Director for the American Association for Organizing Family Social Work, wrote in 1926 about the work of nurses and social workers in rural districts. They both addressed the need for social workers and nurses to provide "family health supervision" and "family case work" (Gamble & Brown, 1926, pp. 276–277). In urban areas, the settlement house brought nursing and social work together to provide these services.

The settlement house movement focused the efforts of these two professions on the problems of the poor, new immigrants, workers, school children, and tenement dwellers (always poor and often new immigrants or transplants from the rural South). Settlement houses literally brought the two professions together because their workers were residents in the neighborhoods they served. Born of human need in the 1880s, settlement houses fostered collaborative relationships that have lessons for nurses and social workers in the 1990s, another era of social chaos.

Social work in settlement houses might be argued to have its modern roots in the principles of social responsibility espoused by the writer Harriet Martineau, by John Ruskin, Thomas H. Green at Oxford, and numerous others. These reformers believed in the social responsibility of the whole for the misery of those less fortunate. In particular, Harriet Martineau directed attention toward the misery of working people. John R. Green and Samuel A. Barnett envisioned charity work among the poor of east London by establishing a settlement house, and Arnold Toynbee inspired the Oxford group to address the problems of the poor. The visions of these social reformers resulted in the establishment of Toynbee Hall in July of 1884 by the University Settlement Association, a committee of Oxford and Cambridge Universities (Holden, 1922). Samuel Coit, an American, went to live at Toynbee Hall in 1886. As a result of his experiences, he and a friend, Charles B. Stover, established the Neighborhood Guild in New York City in 1887, changing its name in 1891 to the University Settlement (Holden, 1922).

Women were clearly in the vanguard of the settlement house effort, although they are not credited with its founding. In fact, 70% of the settlement house heads, as well as residents, were women. "There was . . . what Jane Addams described as a 'subjective necessity' in the founding of the settlements and in the life of community service which women like Ms. Wald undertook" (Brilliant, 1915/1991, p. xii). The settlements were places "for college-educated women who were not content to play out traditional roles of daughter and mother by the hearth at home. Rather, these women wanted to use their training and knowledge for an enlightened purpose, in the spirit of the Progressive Era" (Brilliant, 1915/1991, pp. xii–xiii). Lillian Wald said in a speech to students at Vassar College on October 12, 1915 that "Upon the educated woman evolves the task of readapting the social interests of her sex to a changed physical and spiritual environment" (Wald, 1989, p. 83).

ROLE AND FUNCTION OF THE EARLY SETTLEMENT HOUSES

Some of the original settlement houses established by nurses, social workers, or both were Hull-House (1889) in Chicago; Henry Street Settlement (1893), originally called the Nurses' Settlement, and Uptown Nurses' Settlement (1896) in New York City; Phyllis Wheatley House (1924) in Minneapolis, Minnesota; Potrero Nurses' Settlement (1898) in San Francisco; Gurdon W. Russell Settlement House (1910) established by the Visiting Nurse Association in Hartford, Connecticut; the Nurses Settlement (1900) in Richmond, Virginia; and the South End House in Boston (1891) (Ashe, 1906; Karger, 1986; Minor, 1902; Woods & Kennedy, 1970; Woods, 1898). Settlement houses offered wide varieties of concrete services and philosophies: "organizing neighborhoods into political forces that fought for and obtained such egalitarian advances as child labor laws, public health laws, kindergarten and day care programs" (Loavenbruck & Keys, 1987, p. 557). Specific services such as visiting nursing, public housing, music schools and art programs for the poor, community-based adult education services, courses for naturalization, and parks and playgrounds might be offered. Typically, settlements would champion a cause; once the government sanctioned a program in response, that program would become an independent agency. For example, the visiting nurse service in New York City emerged from the pilot work of Lillian Wald's Nurses' Settlement (Loavenbruck & Keys, 1987, p. 557). Settlements were often at philosophical odds with charity organizations. The latter dispensed relief only to the worthy poor. Settlements did not distinguish among the poor and focused on social reform, tackling the causes of social problems such as substandard housing, child labor, and poverty (Hunter, 1919; Wade, 1967). They created case management, or at least a system that gave birth to case management. "Settlement houses . . . were greatly involved in documenting family, immigrant group, and social and neighborhood problems. The case management system was rudimentary—but effective. It consisted of index card files listing each family's needs and involvements. . . . Early settlement workers were involved in case and service coordination" (Weil & Karls, 1988, p. 4).

Most of the work of the early, formative settlement house was carried out by volunteers, most of them female (Trolander, 1975, p. 26). They were pragmatic, action oriented, and committed to the settlement house philosophy, outlook, and intervention modes. The story of the settlement house workers is also a tale of collaboration between social workers and nurses.

THE SETTLEMENT HOUSE: WOMAN BORN, WOMAN NURTURED, WOMAN POWERED

Social workers and nurses were the founders of many of the early and most prominent and, we might add, extant settlement houses. That their work intertwined was important to the development of each of these predominantly women's professions. It also explains some of the public's confusion between the two. In 1912, Lillian Wald, founder of the Nurses' Settlement in New York City with her colleague Mary Brewster (Wald, 1915), was awarded the Gold Medal of the National Institute of Social Sciences (sponsored by the Rotary Club) to recognize her lifelong service as sociologist, organizer, and publicist (Wald, 1915). Although she was a nurse, Lillian Wald has been described as a social worker by biographers, historians, and early reviewers of her work. So social work stole Lillian Wald from nursing.

Jane Addams, founder with Ellen Gates Starr of Hull-House Settlement in Chicago, frequently stated that social work was a form of sociology (1935). At the time of the founding of Hull-House, formal higher education for social work often took place in sociology departments. So this desire of Addams to link the two fits into the academic context of the now-divided fields. It is also useful to note the male domination of the sociology field, sociologists' avoidance of reform causes to promote themselves as "objective," and the tendency by sociologists to denigrate social work (dominated in its early leadership by women) as less objective and, therefore, academically inferior to sociology. Had Addams' approach prevailed, sociology would be very different (Trolander, 1991, p. 414).

But how could Addams's way have prevailed when social work was literally thrown out of the academy? At the University of Chicago, neighbor to Addams' Hull-House, the following transpired: "That same year (1920), the University of Chicago formed a separate home for the female adjunct faculty in its sociology department by sending them over to its newly created School of Social Studies Administration. The gender segregation of men in sociology and women in social work seemed complete" (Trolander, 1991, p. 414). And while social work was essentially thrown out of the academy, nursing has spent more than a century trying to get into the academy, with its educational origins in the hospital rather than the university (Fondiller, 1986).

The gender wars in the settlement house movement did not cease with the women social workers being banished from the academy at the University of Chicago. Women are said to combine head and heart, fact and feeling, logic and compassion in their decision making and actions (Veeder, 1992). Women's power or ways of winning (that is, marshaling human and material resources to get things done, to effect action) are quite different from those of men, who usually have formal public power, status, and roles. Women are said to use consensus models, to build bridges, to create networks (at times called webs). Indeed, "the settlement house approach to social reform has generally been a cooperative, consensus-building one, utilizing traditional channels" (Trolander, 1982, p. 349). Against this "female" way of operating was cast the Saul Alinsky model in the 1960s. The settlement house movement was transformed by Alinsky and his followers from a liberal-activist and change-agent orientation to conservative, and its consensus-building, peace-keeping use of traditional channels and methods (traditionally female) were rejected. Alinsky asserted that settlement houses were no longer in touch with the neighborhoods, did not know influential community leaders, and did not know what the community really wanted. In short, the settlement houses were unrealistic and, hence, obsolete (Trolander, 1982, p. 349).

The Alinsky (a self-styled radical community organizer) model stressed an adversarial rather than cooperative approach; it stressed conflict and giving the poor the ability to speak and demand for themselves; the poor were pitted against other groups in society. This was a clearly "male" model or approach. The settlement house approach, on the other hand, has promoted a multiplicity of reforms on behalf of low-income people. . . . They have done so by helping to build bridges among different groups of people . . . and they have used these relationships to promote change through cooperation rather than conflict. Settlement houses have shown remarkable durability for an institution with a traditional commitment to reform. Indeed, what is most unique and significant about the settlement houses is their preeminence in the midst of their advocacy for social change. (Trolander, 1982, pp. 362–363)

Just as the settlement house movement, since its founding in the 1880s, has not been isolated from the struggles of society, neither has it been separate from the evolutionary struggles of these two professions. It is not surprising that many of the leaders of both professions were and still are ardent feminists, although social workers appeared to have been more involved than were nurses in the early years. During Sophia Palmer's editorship of the *American Journal of Nursing*, Lavinia Dock, a Henry Street Settlement nurse, wanted the journal to lend its editorial support to the suffrage movement. Miss Palmer maintained that the journal should remain neutral on political issues that had no bearing on nursing (Christy, 1971).

Jane Addams and Dorothea Dix, who was a social reformer and Superintendent of Nurses of the Union Army, have been described as the most modern and feminist women of their time. "Each fashioned a role that was public in its concern with broad social policy but was 'feminine' in that it stressed the values of nurturing and ministering to the unfortunate" (Greenstone, 1979, p. 538). "In short, these women's 'feminine' virtues were especially important in their public careers as reformers" (Greenstone, 1979, p. 531).

Even more than Dix, Addams explicitly stressed the need for a distinctly feminine perspective in reforming almost every facet of American society. . . . By assigning compassion and the nurture of individual capacities to the woman's world of home and family, the culture of Dix and Addams literally domesticated these feminine reform values. (Greenstone, 1979, pp. 531–532)

GROWTH OF THE FAMILY TREE:
DIVERGING BRANCHES

As the settlement house model flourished, so too the professions of nursing and social work grew and developed, sometimes together and sometimes separately. The most significant difference was the path to educational preparation. Social work was firmly rooted in the academe from relatively early in its history. The New York School of Philanthropy, founded in 1898 by the Charity Organization Society as a 6-week summer school was the pioneer for social work education. By 1903 to 1904, the course was an academic year, and by 1910, 2 years (Hollis & Taylor, 1951, p. 9). By 1915, "some fifteen or eighteen schools of social work were in existence" (Bruno, 1957, p. 140). The oldest, in the East, had been organized by practicing social workers, each with a tenuous relationship to a university and preferring to maintain an independent existence. In the Midwest, at the University of Minnesota, Ohio State University, and Indiana University, schools were established as undergraduate bachelor's degree programs. This model was to prevail, for by 1923, the independent schools had each become part of a university (Bruno, 1957, pp. 142–144). When this evolution was accomplished, social workers then sought to make master's degree preparation the entry level for professional practice. Reporting for the Study Committee of the Council on Social Work Education at its annual meeting in 1951, chair Harriett M. Bartlett outlined plans for a generic 2-year master's degree course (Bruno, 1957).

Nursing's path to the academy has been much more uneven. The first training schools were in hospitals, and in 1998 there are still hospital programs to prepare nurses, although their numbers continue to decline. In 1899, the first postgraduate program for superintendents of hospitals and training schools was established at Teachers College, Columbia University (Nutting, 1920). Early in the 20th century, baccalaureate programs were developed (Gray, 1960) followed by master's degree programs for specialty preparation. In the 1990s, we are still struggling with lack of consensus over the bachelor's degree as the entry level (Fondiller, 1986; Pew Health Professions Commission, 1994).

Collaboration continues to be hampered by the discrepancy in education between the two professions and the settings for that education. Whereas social work education takes place in colleges and universities, nurses can acquire their basic preparation, enabling them to sit for state licensure as registered nurses, in a hospital training school, community or junior college, or a 4-year college or university program leading to a bachelor's, master's, or doctoral degree in nursing. Both professions have doctoral degree programs in college and university settings, and many social workers and nurses also have earned doctoral degrees in other fields. The problem of educational disparity is most apparent in clinical settings, where typically the social worker has a master's degree in social work and the nurse a diploma or an associate's, bachelor's, or master's degree, but most often one of the first two, particularly if the setting is a hospital.

Social work and nursing have specialists as well as generalists. The first courses for specialist preparation in nursing were postgraduate non-degree-granting courses. Public health nurses led the way in advanced practice with the creation of postgraduate courses. Charlotte Macleod, former Superintendent of the Waltham Training School in Waltham, Massachusetts, planned and organized the Training School for Nurses of the Boston Instructive District Nursing Association in 1906 (Brainard, 1922). The first formal postgraduate courses for nurse anesthetists were established somewhere between 1909 and 1912 (Bankert, 1989). Specialty preparation in nursing is now usually acquired through a master's degree program, but some postgraduate certificate programs for nurse practitioners and nurse midwives still exist. Social workers can specialize in their master's degree work.

Specialization in social work evolved in several forms. A nurse and a physician began hospital social work at the Massachusetts General Hospital (MGH). Born in Wisconsin and raised in Minnesota, Ida Cannon began her public health nursing career as a visiting nurse for the St. Paul Associated Charities. During this time, she took courses in sociology and psychology at the University of Minnesota and heard Jane Addams speak. She moved to Cambridge to live with her brother and his family to attend the Boston School for Social Workers, later Simmons College School of Social Work, and began volunteer work in the newly established (1905) social services unit at MGH. After graduation in 1907, she joined the staff at MGH and worked with Dr. Richard Cabot, physician for outpatients and administrator of the social services unit, on the evolution of both the social service department and medical social work (Cannon, 1938; Pennock, 1928). Thus, the specialty of medical social work evolved from the work of a nurse who had discovered her interest in social work through her years as a visiting nurse.

Another specialty in social work, psychiatric social work, grew from a shift in philosophy for some social workers from social reform to working on individual adjustment. This shift occurred in the 1920s, when American society was becoming somewhat indifferent to the problems of the poor (Lundblad, 1995). In 1917, Richmond had published *Social Diagnosis*, a text describing the process of social casework. This method became "*the* technique, the badge of professionalism" (Wade, 1967, p. 438). Shortly thereafter, social workers joined other mental health care professionals as "the Freudian frenzy," decrying the pre-Freudian years as sterile and attributing to Freud the possibilities for being an effective profession that was no longer doomed to relief giving and manipulation of the environment (Wade, 1967).

Both professions struggled with issues of professional status, specialization, and standards for education from the early years of the 20th century. The Flexner report, commissioned by the American Medical Association, lambasted social work and nursing, denying that either was or could be a profession. Thus social workers were eager to embrace special techniques that might give them status, as were nurses (Wade, 1967). These struggles contributed in part to the decline of settlement houses and the disappearance of the staff members living in the neighborhoods they served. Wade quoted Sinclair Lewis' *Ann Vickers* in which he ridiculed social settlements, asserting that the staff began to think of themselves as professionals rather than as social explorers or neighbors and were more interested in talking with one another than with the neighborhood leaders (Wade, 1967, p. 440). The nurses most allied with settlement houses, visiting nurses, were also experiencing a shift in their practice. "With fewer immigrants (after World War I), declining death rates from infectious diseases, and the growing centrality of the hospital, the work of the visiting nurse seemed increasingly inconsequential" (Buhler-Wilkerson, 1985, p. 1160).

With the decline in settlement houses, social workers and nurses were deprived of their most important setting for collaboration. Hospitals did employ many nurses and social workers, but the departments were separate, and the opportunities for collaboration had to be made deliberately rather than occurring naturally under the same roof. Many important models of collaboration were created as social workers and nurses tackled new problems together. However, it was not until the War on Poverty of the late 1960s and early 1970s that the two professions were united once more in neighborhood health centers, the offshoots of many settlement houses that had survived the decades or were the result of either zealous health care professionals or neighborhood activists. In these, collaboration was in a way reborn in settings not unlike those where it first began.

In the chapters to follow, we will describe nursing and social work collaboration as it exists on the cusp of the 21st century and as it reflects that born at the turn of the previous century. Through the voices of social workers and nurses, we will take you on a journey through the present and envision the future.

REFERENCES

Addams, J. (1935). *Forty years at Hull-House*. New York: Macmillan.

Ashe, E. (1906). Nurses' settlements in San Francisco. *Charities and the Commons, 16*, 45–47.

Bankert, M. (1989). *Watchful care*. New York: Continuum.

Barton, C. (1912). *The Red Cross in peace and war.* Meriden, CT: Journal Publishing Company.

Brainard, A. M. (1922). *The evolution of public health nursing.* Philadelphia: Saunders.

Brilliant, E. (1991). Introduction. In L. D. Wald, *The house on Henry Street* (pp. i–xxviii). New Brunswick, NJ: Transaction Publishers. (Original work published 1915)

Buhler-Wilkerson, K. (1985). Public health nursing: In sickness or in health? *American Journal of Public Health, 75,* 1155–1161.

Bruno, F. J. (1957). *Trends in social work 1874–1956.* New York: Columbia University Press.

Cannon, I. M. (1938). Changes in hospital care through social service. *Trained Nurse and Hospital Review, 100,* 364–368.

Christy, T. (1971). Equal rights for women: Voices from the past. *American Journal of Nursing, 71,* 288–293.

Fondiller, S. H. (1986). The entry issue: How much longer? An historian's view. *Journal of the New York State Nurses Association, 17*(2), 7–14.

Gamble, L. A., & Brown, J. C. (1926, May 15). Ask a question. *The Survey,* pp. 276–277.

Gray, J. (1960). *Education for nursing—a history of the University of Minnesota school.* Minneapolis, MN: University of Minnesota Press.

Greenstone, J. D. (1979). Dorothea Dix and Jane Addams: From transcendentalism to pragmatism in American social reform. *Social Service Review, 53,* 527–559.

Holden, A. C. (1922). *The settlement idea: A vision of social justice.* New York: Macmillan.

Hollis, E. V., & Taylor, A. L. (1951). *Social work education in the United States.* New York: Columbia University Press.

Hunter, R. (1919). The relation between social settlements and charity organization. In *Twenty-ninth national conference of charities and corrections* (pp. 302–314). Washington, DC: National Association of Charities and Corrections.

Karger, H. J. (1986). Phyllis Wheatley house: A history of the Minneapolis black settlement house, 1924–1940. *Phylon, 47*(3), 79–90.

Lewis, S. (1933). *Ann Vickers.* Garden City, NY: Doubleday, Doran.

Loavenbruck, G., & Keys, P. (1987). Settlements and neighborhood centers. In *Encyclopedia of social work* (18th ed., Vol. 2, pp. 556–561). Silver Spring, MD: National Association of Social Workers.

Lundblad, K. S. (1995). Jane Addams and social reform: A role model for the 1990s. *Social Work, 40,* 661–669.

Minor, M. J. (1902). The nurses' settlement in Richmond, Va. *American Journal of Nursing, 2,* 996–998.

Nightingale, F. (1860). *Notes on nursing: What it is and what it is not.* London: Harrison.

Nutting, M. A. (1920). Twenty years of nursing in Teachers College. *Teachers College Record, 21,* 323–326.

Pennock, M. R. (1928). *Makers of nursing history.* New York: Lakeside.

Pew Health Professions Commission. (1994). *Commission policy papers.* San Francisco: University of California Center for the Health Professions.

Trolander, J. A. (1975). *Settlement houses and the great depression.* Detroit, MI: Wayne State University Press.

Trolander, J. A. (1982). Social change: Settlement houses and Saul Alinsky, 1939–1965. *Social Service Review, 56,* 346–365.

Trolander, J. A. (1991). Hull house and the settlement house movement. A centennial reassessment. *Journal of Urban History, 17*, 414.

Van Blarcom, C. C. (1929). *Obstetrical nursing* (2nd ed.). New York: Macmillan.

Veeder, N. W. (1992). *Women's decision-making, common themes . . . Irish voices.* Westport, CT: Praeger.

Wade, L. C. (1967). The heritage from Chicago's early settlement houses. *Journal of the Illinois State Historical Society, 60*, 411–441.

Wald, L. D. (1915). *The house on Henry Street.* New York: Henry Holt.

Wald, L. D. (1989). New aspects of old social responsibilities. Address to Vassar Students 12 October 1915, reprinted in C. Coss (Ed.), *Lillian D. Wald progressive activist* (pp. 76–84). New York: Feminist Press.

Weil, M., & Karls, J. M. (Eds.). (1988). Historical origins and recent developments. In M. Weil & J. M. Karls (Eds.), *Case management in human service practice* (pp. 1–28). San Francisco: Jossey-Bass.

Whitman, W. (1971). *Specimen days.* Boston: D. R. Godine. (Original work published 1882)

Woodham-Smith, C. (1951). *Florence Nightingale 1820–1910.* New York: McGraw Hill.

Woods, R. A. (Ed.). (1898). *The city wilderness a settlement study by residents and associates of the South End House.* Boston: Houghton Mifflin.

Woods, R. A., & Kennedy, A. J. (Eds.). (1970). *Handbook of settlements.* New York: Arno Press. (Original work published 1911)

CHAPTER 4

Social Workers and Nurses on Collaboration: Findings from a Study

Contemplating the social chaos that led social workers and nurses to create settlement houses, we began to think about the current chaos in health and social welfare. Could we not, we reasoned, examine current collaborative models and explore the possibilities for collaboration afforded to us by this time of chaos. Certainly our foremothers and forefathers had, in a way, used the opportunities given them in a time of crisis in the social and health care fabric of the nation to create new models of care delivery to meet the needs of people. Might the 1990s offer opportunities to nurses and social workers not unlike those of the 1890s and the decades thereafter? From such thinking, we moved on to design and conduct a study to elicit from leaders in social work and nursing their vision of the present chaos and the opportunities it offers.

Our study consisted of in-depth interviews with 33 nursing and social work leaders in 1995–1996.

Through our interviews, we heard about the past, shared stories about the present, and envisioned the future with the social workers and nurses who gave so generously of their time to this study. Theirs are the voices of visionaries and realists who have the skills and knowledge to help both professions realize their dreams together (see Exhibit 10, page 000 for themes from the interviews).

EVOLUTION OF COLLABORATION

Lest we lose what we can learn from the past in our rush toward the future, we asked our participants to describe the heritage of collaboration between nurses and social workers in their practice sites. These settings range from a couple of decades to well over 100 years old, so they represent the full span of time when trained nurses and social workers have existed in U.S. health care.

"It is not a power play about control, but it is that in fact that patients have needs and if we are both very good about what we do then that's the model." These are the words of a social worker participant from an agency with a history of nearly a century of collaboration between social workers and nurses. Several persons talked about an expectation of collaboration, of being taught to be cooperative, not competitive, in their socialization to an agency. One nurse said:

> It's always been there. I don't ever remember working without a social worker or that component. . . . We're together all the time. We refer as many people to social workers as they refer to us in the clinic, whether it be a social worker calling with an AIDS patient that needs intervention for IV therapy or us meeting an AIDS patient that's just coming home from New York to his family to die and we need their help in looking for services for the family or in supporting the family.

And from her social worker collaborator:

> The relationship between social workers and nurses goes way back. Social work has been part of this institution since the 1920s—shortly after the role of social workers in health care evolved, when it really started at MGH (Massachusetts General Hospital) in the early 1900s. . . . Historically . . . (this hospital) was formed by a local group as a charitable organization in the late 1800s; it started as child care for sick kids for mill workers and then kids were abandoned so it became an orphanage. . . . There was always a common focus.

Both nurses and social workers said that they share issues in common and work on them together. In some cases, the leaders of both professions within an agency would agree to collaborate. One social worker explained that the model had always been there (within that agency), though she was not sure how collaborative or effective it has been. The nursing leader of this agency explained that social workers and nurses worked out social contracts with each other (how to treat each other) and did the same with patients and their families, rather than creating a pecking order with the physician at top, as in some practice settings.

One of the community hospitals was among the first to go with a nurse–social worker team approach (almost 15 years ago). The nurse leader in this institution described nurses, social workers, and physicians working together in a triad in the inpatient, subacute, homecare, and community services offered by the hospital. A social worker in a mental health specialty facility described some divergence between the two professions brought about by diagnostic related groups (DRGs) a decade or so ago, and then a struggle and much change over the past 5 years as social workers and nurses were coming together once again. In her view, social workers and nurses come from different orientations (that is why one chooses one or the other profession), but have some core that is similar. The collaboration can be exciting, she said, if both professions can get out of turf guarding. This woman has worked in a variety of settings and described the partnership evident in community mental health centers and how members of the two professions depended on each other in the early days.

The nursing leader of a large teaching hospital medical complex described a history in that institution of nursing being a closed system, alienating social workers, and of a misuse of power in nursing. She said nurses chose to identify with the aggressor, taking power for its own sake. Nurses, in her view, suffered from a lack of role models. Nurses in this hospital believed they were under siege; they got kicked, so they kicked other departments, creating a long, strained relationship. Nursing and social work were working in a parallel manner, not working together. Role clarification was very poor, and there was no sense of collaboration. There were some positive examples in specialties such as the AIDS group practice, in pediatrics, and in the hematology/oncology multidisciplinary team.

In a community-based agency, the social work leader viewed the interface as traditional within traditional roles. She also described enrichment with clinical people, putting a premium on quality and quality care. Among the management team for this agency there is a nurturing role of leaders that sets a tone of collaboration and teamwork, rather than backbiting for turf. A nurse leader in the same community agency described the collaboration as always having been there as a multidisciplinary team in long-term care as dictated by regulations.

A community visiting nurse association (VNA) has a very large nurse to social worker ratio, so collaboration is a small part of the agency functions. A nurse must be involved in a case before social work can be needed; usually at that point, three to four different disciplines are involved, and a formal meeting is necessary to solve the very complex problems.

In a major teaching hospital, the nursing leader described a history of collaboration from the context of the history of the agency. The philosophy of this hospital is not hierarchical, so it lends itself to collaboration among disciplines.

At a community hospital, according to its social work leader, social workers and nurses have been interacting since the 1920s and have been working together on discharge planning for 20 to 25 years, with both disciplines practicing within the same department.

The stories of long-term collaboration were many. Participants described this collaboration thus: it has "always been there"; 12 years of collaboration, working closely together; over a 100-year history of collaboration; collaboration in case management. Sometimes collaboration is the closest in certain units of a large organization. For example, one social worker described collaboration as existing primarily in the external system, working together on discharge planning, the after-care phase, and long-term care. Five years ago in this community medical center, social workers and nurses began to practice case management. Until 1991, social workers and nurses had always been collaborative and now they are true collaborators.

Two social worker–nurse dyads we interviewed were involved in collaborative models designed for the two professions to work together, along with other disciplines, to tackle specific problems. In one of these, both the social worker and the nurse characterized the model as comanagement of a project between social work and nursing that was designed that way. The second team, focusing on families enrolled in an early intervention program, characterized this collaboration as a holistic approach to patient care. Social workers and nurses were supportive of each other in this setting, working together and helping each other.

Often the social work–nursing team was part of a larger team that included physicians. One social worker at a community hospital felt that the relationships between hospitals and physicians are changing, becoming more interdependent rather than hospitals developing standards and dealing with their own disciplines and physicians out there doing their own thing. In her view, physicians are becoming employees of health care networks, so it's an opportunity (for social work and nursing) to finally get that key piece as part of those teams and for the physicians to have to play differently now.

One nurse administrator stated that nurses, social workers, and physicians work as a triad in inpatient, subacute, home care, and the community. She also believed that the nurse and the social worker work more in large group practices with physicians and saw them acting as physician extenders. She felt that the physicians can't afford to spend a lot of time in the hospital making rounds and could have the social worker or nurse serve as case manager for their patients. A social worker stated that the nurses are on the front line working with the physician, and that nurses, doctors, and social workers are all recognized as important jobs at her institution. Representatives from nursing, social work, and physicians meet weekly at interdisciplinary meetings, which improves communication between the team members.

In another institution, the nurse administrator noted that working on collaborative models is almost an expectation, and that the medical community doesn't even know the underpinnings. Another nurse administrator stated that it can be difficult for physicians to see beyond the medical aspects, but the nurse and social worker can. She also felt that the physician puts the patient together as a whole and that this could be a turf issue if someone else were to come along and take over this role. A nurse administrator stated that the social worker and nurse collaborate very closely in a very physician-oriented model in her setting. She continued to state that the social workers and nurses operate as a team, as colleagues, but that it is true of physicians, also. Yet, she has noted an elitist triangulation with the physician to be higher on the hierarchy rather than collaborating, which causes problems at her institution. She believed that medicine feels threatened by the move to the community and that physicians are scared that they have lost control, but not so much with the primary care physicians who see there is no way they can carry everything and don't look down on clinical specialists and social workers, but see the need to be partners. One administrator stated that social workers have a limited role in the medical model, and another that nurses and social workers could be entrepreneurs and hire physicians as needed for their own practices.

The medical model of managed care usually has a physician as the case manager, while the sociomedical model has either a physician, nurse, social worker, or rehabilitation specialist (Schultz, 1991). Regarding the physician in the role of case manager, one social worker stated that there are some physicians who could do it, but that physicians don't want to be in homes and don't know how community agencies work or how families struggle caring for a chronically ill person home. A nurse administrator noted that the physician is part of reasonable discharge planning. Another observed that most physicians are not capable of managing insurance and the social aspects of care.

From long histories of collaboration or relatively new models for working together, the social workers and nurses we interviewed seemed to value past successes and the new challenges presented to them by the chaos of the 1990s. The views were mostly positive, with some negative stories of collaboration, particularly recently under the stresses of downsizing, managed care, and a changing system increasingly driven by third-party payers. Also, stories were mixed on collaboration among social workers, nurses, and physicians. Sometimes the atmosphere of the system as a whole poisoned relationships between professionals, and several participants noted the potential for this phenomenon inherent in the shifting sands of today's health care institutions. In reflecting on the past, our participants could easily identify pluses and minuses of collaboration.

BENEFITS OF COLLABORATION

As these characterizations of the histories of collaboration suggest, both the social workers and nurses in our sample can see benefits of collaboration. Several nurses and social workers allowed that the gray areas between the two professions permit some flexibility in practice and that they had encountered no turf situations.

Many comments were focused on the benefits for patients and their families. These included combining collective talents, meeting the needs of each patient, and seeing what can we do as a team to aid patients. One nurse said:

We can look at the whole family through two different sets of eyes. My background and my training is very strong in physical theory, clinical care, and the social worker's education is more in the social aspects of that care, obviously. Now we've got these two experts—four sets of eyes or two pairs of eyes—looking at one family and giving each other the missing parts of the puzzle. It's a natural collaboration, and we're seeing that in Medicare in total, not only with social work and nursing.

One social worker stated that if nurses and social workers hold to what the patient needs and then look at what each can contribute and where they overlap, the patient's needs can be met. They complement each other; they should not ask a person to be physically and psychically undefended at the same time; nurses can defend one and social workers, the other.

Social workers, according to one member of that profession, see the whole picture, whereas nurses, especially those with associate-degree preparation, are task oriented and do not see the picture outside the institution. Thus, working together, social workers and nurses can focus on what they can do here and what will happen later. As one social worker put it, the social worker brings support and facilitates the next dimension of care, keeping people on a continuum moving the patient toward an increased ability to have (at least some) autonomy. Put another way, patient-centered care is what patients need. The primary motivation is the patient's benefit; social workers are patient advocates and deal with psychosocial issues; nurses deal more with medical concerns. The nurse brings pathophysiology understanding, and the social worker is the synapse with patients about what they are going through, helping them understand how to cope with things. The only real goal, according to one participant, is that of someone going home at the highest level of well-being. Nurses get the patient to the highest possible level and social workers make sure that the home environment is ready. The goal, especially under managed care, is to do the best job in the shortest time. Social workers have knowledge nurses don't and can deal with those issues efficiently. There may be impediments to the patient's recovery. It is the social worker's role to focus on the impediment and facilitate recovery with the nurse. Both work with patients to get the patients home.

According to one social worker, the profession has a role also in helping staff with interpersonal relations within the health care facility; social workers can serve as consultants for nursing interpersonal problems. Nurses and social workers can help each other, sharing case conferences, consulting, collaborating, and communicating with one another. They can create a holistic approach to care, support each other, and take more time with patients. Both can be advocates for patients and see beyond their medical needs. Nurses are in the front lines working with physicians and seeing patients. Social workers know the external community best.

Social workers in hospital settings traditionally had a much more collegial role with physicians than did nurses. The partnership of social workers and nurses in acute care has allowed social workers to provide the broader perspective because nurses in acute care have not been as connected to the community.

The theme of complementary skills and knowledge was expressed not only indirectly through patient goals, but also more directly. Several social workers and nurses described the two very different types of training and the way these come together as an ideal model. Social workers and nurses are interdependent. One can't exist without the other in continuity of care. Both have different orientations and offer different angles on the same issue. Each brings a unique perspective. They can decide together who is the most appropriate person for each role, for example, the case manager. When the focus is on better client care and not on professional self-image, the combination of two world views is dynamite.

The more mature and secure professionals, according to one nurse leader, are less oriented toward power and can begin to relate to the body of knowledge and deal more conceptually with health care delivery systems. The more autonomous the parties, the more collaboration and more respect for each other this partnership will engender. Collaboration can spawn an appreciative acknowledgment of each other's work.

Social workers and nurses agreed that the two professions together provide a holistic approach, a "natural collaboration"; "the best of both worlds—people with training in emotional and mental health and people with training in physical health." Nurses, according to several social workers, are prone to want a quick fix. Social workers help nurses understand human behavior better and realize we can't always cause a change directly.

Overall, our participants painted the portrait of collaboration using mostly bright colors. As one social worker commented: "When you're able to use both (social work and nursing), you really rally the forces and come up with a good package to get the person home, and we've seen that work pretty well." The hues were tempered by the realities of struggling with a cost-driven system, by all the changes imposed by managed care, and by practicing in a complex and problem-fraught society that imposes considerable stress on individuals, families, and communities. But nurses and social workers have much to offer to managed care, too. As one nurse commented: "the stressors that are on families are more fragmented today than they were 20 years ago, and the stressors on the community, the needs to be able to support very ill people at home are much more intense . . . therefore the collaborative approach of nursing and social work is a very essential part to the success of managed care."

In all human interactions there are both pluses and minuses. We asked our participants to comment on any detriments to collaboration that they had experienced in their own practices or among the nurse and social worker teams within their agencies.

DETRIMENTS TO COLLABORATION

Embedded in some of the comments about the positive aspects of collaboration were suggestions that there are also minuses in the relationships. Our participants shared freely of their perceptions of these as well. One nursing leader said that both social workers and nurses are fabulous practitioners, but that business types are needed too. Both professions can benefit from the skill development needed to become full partners. Several social workers and nurses spoke of the conflicts their professions experience with other members of the team, particularly psychologists, especially in psychiatric mental health practice.

The gray areas can be detriments to collaboration as well as benefits. Several participants spoke of the not always perfectly clear boundaries, and one gave the example of a social worker being unable to contact the

VNA about discharge planning. She suggested that such turf issues are best worked out by the team and not through a directive.

The pay differentials between social workers and nurses in certain agencies and institutions were a problem. So were the differences in education. One social service administrator said it was frustrating for social workers to compare 2 years of education to become a registered nurse versus 6 years of preparation for social work. It was different, she said, working with nurses with bachelor's and master's degrees. Numbers of social workers compared to nurses can also be a problem in agencies. When there are many more nurses than social workers, it is harder to work in teams or have close collaboration; the social workers need to spread themselves too thinly and don't have time to develop the collaborative relationships that would be ideal.

Schedules, too, are detrimental to collaboration. One nurse executive described the scenario in hospitals: nurses are divided into 3 8-hour shifts 7 days a week, and social workers are on a 9-to-5 Monday-through-Friday schedule with no weekend coverage. These differences in schedules lead to difficulties in communication. This same nurse executive pointed out that her hospital has no electronic record-keeping system, making for complex communications between professionals who have divergent schedules. The logistic difficulties can lead to lack of face-to-face interactions. Other participants pointed out that communication needs to be crystal clear. One social worker said that nurses could shut out social workers with lingo. Both professions can suffer because of lack of a common language and a lack of understanding of macro health issues.

Social workers and nurses fear change. Both feel forced to change because of money, and it doesn't feel good. Some nurses are resistant to change and want control in the view of social workers. Both professions have high anxiety about the future and fear competition in the face of a lack of job security and role ambiguity. Some social workers see problems with nurses as case managers and leaders of the team, believing that social work becomes more fuzzy then. Some see duplication in what they and nurses do, particularly in the psychosocial aspects of care, and experience frustration at having no tangible task, as nurses have. Social workers fear losing status if nurses are to be in control of a managed care system in and out of the hospital. Decreased length of stay for patients is detrimental to collaboration. Cultural change occurs for both professions as the acuity level of care they are administering increases. There is frustration on the part of social workers who perceive they have little or no role in health care changes. The care delivery system does not always support social workers, leading to elimination of these providers. On the other hand, there are barriers to keep them from doing each other's jobs. There is resistance to bringing social workers into the community (home care agencies) and to psychiatric mental health nurses in the community as well.

One nurse questioned the philosophical match between the two professions. Nurses lack understanding of cultural issues and are unfriendly to persons of different cultures, according to one social worker's view. Social workers are better than nurses with persons with HIV. How then, can the two collaborate?

Nursing's self-esteem seems more fragile. Nurses need to make the transition from locus of control when in the community and recognize who is really in charge—the client. They see patients as segmented and not as a whole. Nurses have to learn when to let clients do for themselves and how much to be directly involved in clients' problems.

Nurses try to do everything, to be rescuers. Furthermore, nurses are uncomfortable with ambiguity and see things as black and white, whereas social workers see things as gray. Nurses may feel social workers aren't doing their job because the problems aren't fixed. Nurses tend to be reactive and social workers are trained to be nonreactive.

Social workers are well grounded conceptually, but cannot always operationalize in practice. They feel like the low persons on the hierarchy in hospitals. The underpinnings of two lesser professions in the eyes of others are still there for both social work and nursing.

The minuses in collaboration can be summed up in the comment of one social worker.

> People feel threatened in this managed care climate. . . . Nurses traditionally saw acute care as the place to be in terms of giving credibility or proving your skill set. The environment has now shifted, and truly the future is now home care and subacute units, but for those who are in acute care, to talk about moving to a nursing home is tough to swallow—a very bitter transition. So you see nursing trying to hang onto anything in the acute care setting . . . for example, case management positions.

So what can be done about the minuses for collaboration? There is a need to look at where to pull apart and where to pull together, and to use the creative tension between the two professions and capitalize on the cultures within the professions. One person suggested combining forces through our professional organizations. Because change is happening all around, the opportunity exists to create new models of care to meet the needs of the public and demonstrate that nurses and social workers can make a difference. Measuring outcomes is one way to concretely demonstrate that we can make a difference together.

MEASURING OUTCOMES

There was consensus among the participants about the need to measure outcomes, and there were many ideas about data to collect. Both professions have measurable goals toward which they direct their energies. Social workers suggested looking at where patients go after discharge from an acute care or step-down facility. One can ask whether patients can care for themselves. What is the level of patient functioning; are they able to perform usual activities of daily living, go back to work, attend school, and so on? Is the patient in a stable social system environment? What behavioral changes can be observed in a patient? What are the rates of readmissions to acute care, the number of emergency department visits, and the length of stay in inpatient facilities? What are the infection rates, rates of deep vein thrombosis, and comorbidities? How is the pain management? They could develop pain scales (subjective measures) together. In specialty practices, outcome measures are easier to develop. For example, in developing collaborative models to care for children with developmental delays, one can measure developmental milestones. Reaching pregnant women through outreach programs and drawing them into care, one can measure prenatal outcomes such as birthweight and gestational age. In a model for pregnant women using drugs, the social worker–nurse team evaluates pregnancy outcomes and whether the women stop substance use.

Some participants gave specific examples. One social worker noted: "Of all of the indicators, we're paying real close attention to patients that come back in, and we can set thresholds and if you send somebody home with homecare." Another social worker gave the example of a person who had a stroke and asked whether the expectation would be that the person walk and talk at the end of the rehabilitation program, how the person would get there, what the person would need to do each day—using these as goals and then putting together the care to meet the goals.

Other outcome measurement could be designed to examine patient satisfaction with services and the satisfaction of other consumers such as families. What is the level of patient satisfaction with such factors as being on time? Are the patients' needs satisfied by their definitions? Are physicians satisfied with the outcomes of programs designed and implemented by social workers and nurses?

Outcome evaluation can occur at the system's level as well. Nurses and social workers suggested examining how successful a scheme of triaging is; what services are providers reimbursed for; and within managed care, who is the least expensive provider. How many days was a patient denied access to a placement out of the acute care setting? Did social work or nursing variables contribute to the placement denial? If social workers are not available for weekend discharge, does this contribute to prolonging a more expensive level of care?

Some participants suggested looking at health and not just disease, working together to determine measurements, including psychological outcomes. If one can define what one is trying to achieve—working with clients as to what they want to achieve—then maybe one can plan how to get those results. Care maps or critical pathways are being created in many settings. These might help us to profile high risk profile patients then target them for in-depth interface work. However, as one social worker cautioned, goals take time to achieve in social work and that social work is not a product.

Many of our participants stressed the need for the two professions to work together. Several pointed out the need to evaluate together and not attribute outcomes to any one profession or group. All seemed concerned about the need to measure outcomes in some way to satisfy the payers, and that managed care seems focused on concrete outcomes and not on the softer, less measurable aspects of caring that are so much a part of social work and nursing. A sense of urgency and perhaps fear seemed to characterize the responses to this question.

Outcomes relate to the reasons patients choose providers of health care. If given the luxury of choosing at all, they talk with others about which physician has the best results from plastic surgery, the fewest cesarean sections, or is amenable to vaginal birth after cesarean section. Nurses and social workers, until recently, have been the more invisible among health care professionals, hidden as they have been as employees of hospitals, nursing homes, and long-term care facilities. Only in home care and other community settings have they been more, or even the most, visible of health care professionals. With a return to community-based care, they have an opportunity to be visible providers and encourage direct access for consumers to a variety of health care professionals. After all, they can be contractors with managed care systems as well as physicians and hospitals are.

DIRECT ACCESS BY PATIENTS
TO HEALTH CARE PROVIDERS

As we contemplate a future with managed care, capitation, or whatever systems evolve out of the present chaos, many hope that the concept of a gatekeeper will mature from that of an individual group of providers (physicians) or third-party payers, to an open system in which patients can choose whom to visit based on individual needs and goals. Our participants envisioned anything from a very closed to an open system. One nurse executive recalled a voucher system being tried that allowed the employee access to whomever the employee chooses. A social worker suggested that most physicians are not capable of managing social aspects of care; that patients need direct access to these services. Several feared that as gatekeepers, physicians will keep them out. The optimists among the group saw changes, envisioned partnerships between nurses and social workers, and believed that they can work together to recommend services, envisioning many untapped opportunities under managed care. It may be that the payer will justify the need for service and not dictate by whom that service will be delivered. Service may become tied more to reimbursement and less to the provider system. One participant pointed out that under capitation, providers get to keep more money if they keep patients well. The best and most cost effective caregiver may not be the physician; the payment structure needs to change. In regard to the ownership of team practices, one social worker believed that everyone involved could buy shares and that the practices can't be just physician owned. The wave of the future, according to a nurse administrator, is that physician groups can become their own health maintenance organizations without directly paying 20% to the managed care company for the overhead and billing or dispensation of the capitated rate.

One social worker interviewed believed that access to providers may break down with physicians in control. A nurse administrator stated that the physicians hold all capitated dollars and make all decisions regarding whom to use. A social worker interviewed stated that access for clients to the providers is going to be hard to get because as physicians begin to be gatekeepers, they will keep nursing and social workers out. They are worried about their incomes and members of their profession's incomes and they don't want nurse practitioners in practice because of the expense. Another nurse administrator believed that access depends on the oversupply of physicians, the changes in medical students (less a "me generation"), and the changes in specialties chosen.

In psychiatric mental health care systems, social workers and nurses could collaborate with physicians on telephone calls to patients. They could break from the 50-minute visit model to shorter visits just to see how people are doing. In fact, this is already happening in some settings.

Many participants expressed optimism, stating that experiences with open patient access have been positive. In the views of some, including social workers and nurses working in health maintenance organizations, these managed care systems give patients access to and the tools for home care. There is a growing demand by patients for a greater role in their care.

The nurse in a focused collaborative program argued for more access: "one-stop shopping in health care," especially for high-risk clients. Patients might choose a system of care for the range of services it provides rather than searching for individual providers for different needs.

Those less optimistic pointed out that primary care is a difficult role for nurse practitioners, as they often can't make referrals due to cost. Some believe access is getting harder. Providers have incentives to do less today. Many VNAs and other home care agencies must rely on physicians as gatekeepers and home care intakes from physicians and believe that there should be direct access for patients to home care services.

Overall, participants expressed some pessimism about patients even having choices about care or health care providers under managed care or capitated schemes. Certainly the menu is shrinking for employees as employers move to cut costs of health care coverage. The more optimistic envisioned opportunities for new models of care and access, particularly if outcomes can be demonstrated that save costly time in acute care settings. Such discussion led us to ask our participants to share their concepts of an ideal system of collaboration.

COLLABORATION BETWEEN NURSES AND SOCIAL WORKERS: IMAGINING THE IDEAL

Social workers and nurses would be direct carriers of services in an ideal system. For example, patients could go directly to nurse practitioners and then be triaged to other services as needed. Social workers and nurse practitioners together could establish primary care practices, particularly in pediatrics and in an obstetrics and gynecology primary care model. Social workers and nurses could create a system of case management for a broad community of patients. Case managers could function as physician extenders to protect the quality of and access to care. They could consider food and transportation, housing and social concerns, consolidating these and other health care needs. Nurses and social workers now run long-term care facilities and home health care agencies—why not other types of facilities? In home care services, roles of social workers and nurses could run across the care continuum; these providers could act as resource coordinators. For a truly interdisciplinary team, both could go on home visits together. All health care needs could be met at one site for selected patient groups. The setting should be dignified; there should be separate women's services from the men's. Some saw the settlement model as ideal.

One managed care system contracting with a community hospital requests a social worker on each of their patients. The nurse executive in this hospital suggested that nurses and social workers could contract with physician groups and managed care systems directly to provide services to their enrollees.

In an ideal model, the focus would be on patient needs instead of what a health care provider is trained to do. Providers would decide who is best equipped to do what for the patient. The case manager[1] or health care manager would be the best person to evaluate the needs of a patient and coordinate services; the case manager could change with the patient's needs. The question would be who offers the skills needed based on assessment of patients, activities of daily living, and so on. In the view of a nurse executive in a community hospital, a collaborative system to get together as a group of providers and disperse as needed for an individual case is needed. Both professions could offer coordination among settings, a circle of care. They could work with physicians to establish a referral system. One social worker cited the ideal collaborative team as the social worker and the advanced practice nurse.

Several models exist that our participants considered ideal. At one large teaching hospital, social workers and nurses created a coordinated care program to keep frail elderly persons at home. Social workers and nurses at a community hospital have one department, not two, for discharge planning and home care. A community health center runs an early intervention program for families; the key players are nurses and social workers. A community hospital has a new families program that is available postpartum. Some of these models focus on prevention as well as early intervention.

Our participants, social workers and nurses in leadership positions, infused us with their energy and enthusiasm for their imagined futures of collaboration. They reminded us of the leaders of the late 19th century who dared to dream a new profession (social work), new models of care when there were no jobs in hospitals (nurses), and specialties (medical social work, public health nursing). Focusing on the needs of the public (immigrants, the poor, the sick) in the places where they lived (tenements, cities, rural areas), worked, played, went to school, and worshiped, they created collaborative models of care delivery, seldom forgetting for whom they were privileged to provide care. In a public health model, they lowered infant and maternal mortality and morbidity rates with prenatal care and well-baby clinics, welcomed and helped integrate immigrants into American life, lowered injury and fatality rates in factories, and raised attendance rates in schools. Health promotion and disease prevention are central to the practice of social workers and nurses.

---

[1]One social work director pointed out that no one wants to be a case, and no one wants to be managed, so maybe we need different language.

PREVENTION AND A NEW COLLABORATION

As the federal government moves toward a medical model in its goal of preventive care for all, social workers and nurses should create systems to manage people in the workplace and the home, helping them manage stress to keep them well. One nurse executive went on to describe a system of computer access for elderly persons through the telephone and monitoring them by keeping in touch through cable television. In the psychiatric services of one community hospital, there is currently a reimbursement experiment for phone calls by providers to prevent emergency department visits and inpatient stays. Through telephone contact, providers can check in with patients and, when needed, do crisis management over the phone to allay the crisis. If we had information systems on line, she said, patients would not have to repeat information and providers could field telephone calls to avert crises.

Providers would refer persons into services and keep people away through prevention. The goal would be to keep people out of acute care settings. If hospitalization became necessary, there would be more case management beyond the hospital and on a continuum. Social workers and nurses could work together in schools, the welfare system, and out in the community.

Social workers and nurses could share the burden of responsibility for patients (such as a suicidal patient), rather than bearing the burden as solo practitioners. They could work together to develop early intervention programs for a variety of groups of patients, not just infants, and models like Head Start. Nurses in hospitals could rotate from inpatient care to outpatient care, and there could be models of collaboration in outpatient care to focus on prevention. Through all of these ideas runs the thread of the need for diversity in providers to reach patients and to teach and integrate cultural sensitivity through all systems. Part of this sensitivity would include recognition of complementary (alternative) systems of health care.

COMPLEMENTARY THERAPIES, SYSTEMS, AND PROVIDERS: A NEW AGE

Our participants in general agreed that patients are fearful about telling health care providers of their use of complementary systems and therapies. The creation within the National Institutes of Health of the Mind–Body Institute lends some legitimacy to complementary therapies and therapists. In the view of one nurse executive, however, we need champions in medicine to give credibility to these. The question is, in the words of one social work director, "Do alternative therapies find their home in the health professions"? Whatever the answer, how can we measure outcomes? We need to do empirical studies to show what works before we adopt strategies. Some of the social workers and nurses we interviewed believed we must mix Eastern and Western health care to meet the needs of patients. They pointed out a need to work with other healers for better health care and noted that nurses and social workers can facilitate this process. As providers with a holistic view, we can look at how what is going on makes the person feel and accept anything that helps as long as it is not in conflict and bring in these therapies as adjunct to (Western medicine) treatment. We need to incorporate an Eastern philosophy of healing with the Western view. There are alternative healers in place within health maintenance organizations already. One participant said that the following therapies can be very important in helping persons with substance abuse problems: acupuncture, spiritual healers, therapeutic touch, stress management, relaxation, nutrition, and vitamin supplements. The best approach in substance abuse is not the medical approach.

The effects of having physicians as team members on attitudes toward complementary therapies varied according to one nurse administrator. She stated that physicians were generally not available on weekends. Her institution has physicians on staff with lots of Eastern thinking, so they have a balance between alternative and medical modalities. One social worker stated that alternative therapies will be very controversial in physician-dominated settings. One nurse administrator was told by a physician that the reason health care costs are so high is because nurses and social workers are out there with alternative therapies so medicine has to step back in. Another stated that patients are fearful to tell primary care providers of the use of alternative systems.

Some participants urged caution in embracing complementary therapies. Part of our responsibility as health care professionals is to assure that our patients don't become victims. Payment for this care is a problem, so patients might be deprived of help. One community hospital is located in a conservative community; in the social worker's view, patients don't ask about complementary therapies and probably won't.

In an increasingly diverse practice environment, we probably cannot ignore the role of complementary therapies in the care our clients are seeking. Although the need to incorporate or at least acknowledge these therapies will vary from community to community, they will play an increasingly important role in the total care package. With the creation of the Office of Alternative Medicine within the National Institutes of Health in 1992 (Rubik, 1995), considerable legitimacy was lent to therapies once considered outside the Western medicine circles in the United States.

We have a heritage of caring for the whole person, the family constellation, and the community, often incorporating complementary therapies. Social workers and nurses in settlement houses learned about the healing practices immigrants brought from their countries of origin. Current interest in these practices offers new opportunities for collaboration among health care professionals.

OPPORTUNITIES FOR COLLABORATION

Nurses and social workers can be entrepreneurs and establish private practices, hiring physicians as needed. They could work in large group practices with physicians and serve as case managers to keep people out of hospitals or move them in and out quickly. There are models now in psychiatric mental health practices, such as the program at one community hospital, for collaboration on intensive care cases among social workers, nurses, and physicians.

In oncology and hospice care, they can serve as advocates for patients with physicians so the social network can absorb the patients' needs. Nurses can predict the trajectory across the continuum; help plan in-home care and for future admissions. In primary care, they could run clinics and centers and use physicians for referrals. They can see patients and families together in the community to talk about goals.

Nurses and social workers could be an unbelievable team in the managed care market. They could locate out in the community—it would be too expensive in hospital settings. They could also practice together in behavioral and mental health facilities, in school-based programs, long-term care with elderly persons, in subacute care, and whole-disease management. Nurses and social workers could set up screening in the community. A program for colorectal screening could be set up at a grocery store along with coupons for high fiber foods. They could get in on capitation schemes. For all of these to happen, both professions need to be culturally competent and educate the community, acting as liaisons between Western medicine and immigrant healing practices. They could create patient learning centers. Nurses and social workers could provide outreach to community health centers that are not freestanding by contracting with them for services; create executive health programs; and address domestic violence, drugs, alcohol, smoking, and terminal illness, taking the lead in creating new models. School-based clinics, women's centers, and daycare centers for children and adults offer new and revisited opportunities for collaboration.

One participant urged a stop to whining about what managed care is doing. It is time to stop reeling under managed care and begin to say "let's all take charge." Social workers and nurses should embrace the power they have together. The forced collaboration under managed care and capitation schemes could create equal opportunities for both professions.

Participants are creating and dreaming about new models of care and of collaboration. In the interviews, they reflected a cautious optimism about the opportunities for collaboration and urged abandoning victim behavior and seizing the power that is nursing and social work's together. As the largest groups of health and welfare professionals, there is political and social power, as well as a loyal public among patients and clients. To use this power, however, nurses and social workers need to address the issues that divide them and do some housekeeping within their respective professions.

ISSUES FOR THE PROFESSIONS

Participants willingly shared issues and concerns with us. One social work director queried how to keep each profession sharp so that no one becomes enmeshed and mediocre, how to stay on the cutting edge. How can education reinforce that working together is important and that care(ing) is important? One nurse executive suggested the use of models of supervision from social work in nursing. Both professions might look at the career plans of the members of the units for which they have responsibility. Problems of gender dynamics in nursing and in social work remain; men continue to rise quickly to the top disproportionately to their numbers, as they are the minority of social workers and nurses.

Most case management is learned through continuing education and such preparation is not organized in academia. It is hard to move ahead in New England, one social worker commented, because traditions are deeply rooted. Another social worker explained that traditional social work roles are gone; social work education needs to prepare for today's world. It is harder to develop roles if students are not taught these roles. In the opinion of one nurse executive, most nurses don't know what is going on. More education for the professionals about managed care is needed.

Both professions could be educated together, revamping both social work and nursing education to set the stage for going out in the world. Education is too rigid, especially social work preparation. Social workers have to be aggressive as a profession. Social work has a problem with aggression; usually its practitioners are passive and insecure, according to one social worker participant.

Finally, from the system's perspective as well as that of individual professionals, attention must be paid to spiritual needs of clients, the focus of care placed on wellness and health and keeping people out of the hospital, alternative modalities looked at, and nurses and social workers must be proactive and not reactive. Nurses and social workers should be compensated better in managed care systems and provide quality care at a lower cost.

The theme of being proactive rather than reactive was both overt and covert in the concerns about both professions. Because they often care for victims, perhaps they sometimes adopt victim behavior. As professions with a preponderance of women, they have been disadvantaged in this society and sometimes confuse disadvantage with limitation. The limits on opportunities cannot be blamed on the environments in which they practice; they can create limits within their own ranks that become insurmountable barriers if allowed to do so. Or they can seize the opportunities inherent in the chaos that characterizes health care delivery at present.

CONCLUSIONS

The willingness of our participants to share their opinions, assessments, thoughts, and dreams has created a collage of collaboration between social workers and nurses (see Exhibit 11, page 212 for list of participants). In the chapters that follow, we will explore models of collaboration that work, detail a new model, and challenge the stereotype of downtrodden women's professions. Together, nurses and social workers have the power and abilities necessary to create a revolution in health care delivery for the 21st century similar to that created for the 20th century through the settlement houses and other community-based models of care. In the next chapter, we will present a model for collaboration generated from the data and from the literature.

REFERENCES

Rubik, B. (1995). The NIH office of alternative medicine: What has it accomplished in its 3 years? *Alternative Health Practitioner, 1*, 7–11.
Schultz, P. R. (1991). Managed care. *Washington Nurse, 21*, 16–17.

CHAPTER 5

The Biopsychosocial Individual and Systems Intervention Model: A Model of Collaboration, Coordination, and Accountability

The proposed model for nurse–social work collaboration is called the Biopsychosocial Individual and Systems Intervention Model (BISIM). This model derives from a combination of the most workable interdisciplinary collaboration models at the organizational and administrative levels and a broadly conceived case management intervention approach on individual and small systems (family and other small reference groups) levels. The proposed collaboration model responds to new developments in both nursing and social work education and practice, as well as to current and future developments in managed care noted in both professions' literature. It also mirrors findings from the nurse and social work administrators and practitioners study reported in chapter 4.

INTERDISCIPLINARY COLLABORATION MODELS

Managed care has mandated the collaborative model of professional, interdisciplinary interaction to better serve health and behavioral health consumer groups. This stance has been confirmed by the rapid growth, in both the public and private health and human services sectors, of

> partnerships, alliances, joint ventures, consortia, and networks. . . . Interdisciplinary collaboration in health and mental health social work practice has taken on increasing importance in light of changes in federal and state policies that have emphasized cost controls, the reduced use of institutional care, and the decreased autonomy of physicians. Such changes have made

56

the social work role more central and have created incentives for all groups of professionals to work collaboratively to deliver better coordinated and more efficient care. (Abramson & Rosenthal, 1995, p. 1479)

Although the study of collaboration as an interprofessional activity is fairly new, it is increasingly being seen as a focal issue in the delivery of managed care health services. This is particularly because managed care systems stress coordination as opposed to expensive fragmentation and interdisciplinary services delivery based on both joint service delivery protocols and outcome evaluations in highly complex health and behavioral health situations needing a variety of simultaneous professional interventions (Saltz & Schaefer, 1996).

Collaborative efforts vary greatly. However, they display commonalties in both development and evolution, namely, they all "require certain conditions, commitment, contributions, and competence, and all inherently experience dynamic tensions, which must be expected and managed" (Abramson & Rosenthal, 1995, p. 1481). Collaboration between professions has both advantages and disadvantages. That the advantages far outweigh the disadvantages in no way minimized the necessity for understanding, and resolving wherever possible, the negative effects on consumer service that may result from the actual or potential negatives in interdisciplinary collaboration.

ADVANTAGES TO INTERPROFESSIONAL COLLABORATION

Advantages to collaboration are:

- Inclusion of multiple perspectives and stakeholders; the service delivery "product" will reflect a widely informed and complete point of view.
- Broad and comprehensive analysis of complex and interconnected individual, group, organizational, and community situations improves solutions and intervention responses.
- Inclusiveness promotes a wide base of intervention plan ownership and increased strength for joint implementation of the intervention plan.
- Broader understanding of both consumer and client needs and resources, which leads to improved problem definition and individual intervention and programmatic designs and implementations occurs.
- Improved coordination and service linkages occur.
- Collaborating professionals can factor out those unique skills they possess, concentrate on them, and thereby improve the strength of the team's efforts.

- Sharing as equals can prevent the burnout that is inherent in continuously complex and high stress situations.
- Collaboration is a specific strategy of strength in addressing large institutional processes, be they institutional racism, medical system inaccessibility and cultural insensitivity, or insurer myopia.
- Collaboration enables strong advocacy legislatively, in the media, and with the general public, thus enabling participation in social and economic change in the health and behavioral health care delivery system.

DISADVANTAGES AND OBSTACLES TO INTERPROFESSIONAL COLLABORATION

Considerable attention has also been paid in the literature to potential negatives in interprofessional collaboration. They may include the following:

Unequal actual or perceived power and status differentials exist among members of the collaborating team. If a physician is present, as is frequently the case, the physician is usually assumed to be the titular team leader (Sheppard, 1992). Historically and operationally, however, both nurses and social workers have done the bulk of the leading in direct patient care, regardless of the setting.

Difficulties in achieving equality occurs among different professionals. This is particularly true when physicians are members, even largely titular members, of the interdisciplinary team. Professional perceptions play a crucial role here. In a study of perceived professional competence among psychologists, psychiatrists, and social workers by a group of peer raters (including nurses), perceptions were that professionals sharing the rater's own professional affiliation were more helpful, expert, and warm, as well as the preferred recipient of referrals (Koeske, Koeske, & Mallinger, 1993). Clinical social workers were rated highest on warmth by all raters, but lowest on preferred referral recipient by all raters.

Inequities and communication difficulties arise due to differences in race, gender, culture, and class. Communication issues, which can be exacerbated by actual or perceived differences of any kind, have been noted to be crucial impediments to interdisciplinary collaboration (Abramson & Mizrahi, 1996a, b).

Turf issues exist. Professions such as nursing and social work, both of which have long struggled for professional definition, viability, and autonomy, are not only prone to come into conflict with other professional groups, but with each other. This is particularly true in competitive managed care systems where nurses and social workers are directly competing for dollars, as well as status and prestige.

A further complicating turf issue, resulting from managed care's dictates and highlighted in such crucial nurse–social worker collaborative areas as home health care, is that social work is, by definition, a dependent profession in a system where social work services cannot be billed as free-standing services, but must always be under the umbrella of nursing or medicine. Because social work has few, if any, protocols for its own delivery, it must rely on being "triggered" by another profession's protocols, rather than by its own protocols, as is nursing.

There is poor definition of roles and responsibilities. Some interdisciplinary teams try to head off problems by blurring roles and sharing all tasks and responsibilities equally. This usually dilutes unique-to-profession contributions and confuses both consumers and other professional collaborators. Conversely, there can be role definition that is too narrow rather than blurring. For example, social workers may be perceived by other team members as only taking care of concrete services such as housing, nursing home placements, finances, and support services at home, whereas they perceive themselves as clinician-intervenors in the realm of psychosocial pathology.

Conversely, social workers may assume a great deal more knowledge and sophistication in these clinical areas on the part of other team members (nurses, physicians, and others such as nutritionists and physiotherapists) than in fact exists. Interprofessional role expectations studies have shown that one of the most difficult social work roles for other disciplines to accept is the one that focuses on the person-in-environment (Cowles & Lefcowitz, 1992, p. 192). This, of course, is precisely the area in which social workers are best trained.

The picture may be further complicated by the fact that nursing is trying to acquire more status and dominance in the health and behavioral health care relationship with the consumer. In their attempt to give up their lesser status activities such as cleaning up after physicians and restocking supplies, nurses have sought more discretion and autonomy in the patient psychosocial realm, with the corollary that nurses have become increasingly involved in broader psychosocial interventions with individuals, groups, and communities. These successful strivings and broadening of roles, of course, put nurses on a collision course with social workers, who have long held the psychosocial clinical intervention area as their own (if shared, it is with the other psychological professions, which did not, until the 1940s, include nursing) (Carlton, 1984; Kulys & Davis, 1987).

Different disciplines do not necessarily share the same values or terminologies and may define goals of service and expected service outcomes, and how to measure them, differently. Differences between nursing having protocols or critical pathways for almost every treatment contingency

(Beyea, 1996; Hawkins, Roberto, & Stanley-Haney, 1997; Rawlins & Heacock, 1993) and social work's almost total lack of protocols or critical pathways for treatment episodes illustrate this point dramatically. Another example is differences in defining what the problem is in a given case. For example, nonpsychiatric nurses may be unfamiliar with certain psychosocial or psychiatric diagnostic taxonomies (see chapter 7 for a discussion of diagnostic category issues for the interdisciplinary team); physicians may not know what community resources are available and when and under which circumstances these might be appropriately utilized; and social workers may be unfamiliar with medical diagnosis and treatment and how the course of a physical illness might impact the individual or family, both physically and psychologically (Lee, 1980). Value differences have been largely studied between social work and medicine (Roberts, 1989).

Communication problems may arise due to the setting, acculturation differences among professions, and interpersonal issues.

Inability to deal directly with conflict, "whether organizational, interorganizational, interprofessional, or interpersonal in nature, is perhaps the most critical obstacle to effective collaboration" (Abramson & Rosenthal, 1995, p. 1483). Conflict may be caused by any of the above and more (Mizrahi & Abramson, 1985; Sands, Stafford, & McClelland, 1990). Social work, in particular, is a profession that has great difficulty dealing with conflict and confronting differences. This may pose particular problems in nurse–social worker interaction as professional equals because traditionally both professions are hierarchically bound to lower status positions and female dominated. Neither training or subsequent professional experiences have shown either profession that to address conflict head-on, to think competitively, or to attempt resolution in an entrepreneurial and risk-taking manner can lead to more creative solutions and optimal outcomes (Lowe & Herranan, 1978, 1981).

WHAT NURSES AND SOCIAL WORKERS BRING TO THE COLLABORATION MODEL

Both nurses and social workers are, both by training and predilection, capable of significant contributions to collaboration.

> As an interactive process that synthesizes and integrates the skills, expertise, and resources of individuals to accomplish a goal, collaboration is characterized by interpersonal valuing that changes the relationship and forms a foundation for future interactions. Advance practice nurses contribute to the development of organizational cultures that foster interdisciplinary col-

laboration because of their advanced knowledge, skill, and clinical competence, which contributes to the development of collaborative relationships. (Stichler, 1995, p. 53)

Similarly, for social workers,

Collaboration is a highly effective approach to service delivery, capable of resolving previously intractable problems and creating innovative and comprehensive interventions. The expertise and interaction of the diverse participants combine to produce an unusually deep and rich set of otherwise unattainable resources. Collaborations can be powerful tools for social workers and have many possible applications. Social workers' clinical wisdom can be a great help in the formulation of collaborative strategies and the facilitation of group processes. Social workers need to appreciate the potential of collaboration and to value and maximize their special contribution to this form of practice. (Abramson & Rosenthal, 1995, p. 1486)

Social workers bring core skills to the collaborative mix such as interpersonal communication, social network development, and group facilitation (Andrews, 1990).

Both nurses and social workers are trained to work on collaborative teams. The predominant role in both professions is not that of independent clinician or agent, but collaborator. Tremendous role and status differentials exist between physicians and nurses and social workers (Berger et al., 1996). A good deal has been written, therefore, about nurse-physician problems in collaboration (Koeske, et al., 1993; Lowe & Herranen, 1978, 1981; Sands, et al., 1990; Sheppard, 1992). More recently, the literature speaks to social worker-physician collaborative issues as well (Abramson & Mizrahi, 1996a, b; Azzarto, 1992; Dane & Simon, 1991; Frangos & Chase, 1976; Koeske, et al., 1993; Lowe & Herranen, 1978, 1981; Mizrahi & Abramson, 1985; Netting & Williams, 1996; Roberts, 1989; Sands, 1989; Sands, et al., 1990; Sheppard, 1992).

Issues in collaboration between unequals (at least in the eyes of the dominant professional, usually the physician, but in practice areas such as home health care, also the nurse) cause problems of role, status, leadership, and decision-making differentials. However, when the playing field is leveled to include two professions, nursing and social work, which are more similar in status, the problems do not magically evaporate. Rather, the competition for status between the two may be heightened, as may the squabbles about who does what best, given perceived and actual similarities in training.

For example, nurses may have notions or biases that social workers pollute their relationships with clients. Worse yet, some nurses believe (and more than a few have actually experienced) that cases become unduly complicated, indeed, get much worse, after the social worker comes on the scene. Social workers, for their part, frequently think that nurses approach cases too simplistically and concretely and fail to take into account the psychosocial factors that invariably determine the ultimate health goal, compliance with medical treatment.

Nonetheless, the future for nurse–social work collaboration looks much brighter because of, not despite, shared values and training. The crucial issue becomes the skill level of both nurse and social worker. The higher the skill level of the social worker, for example, the higher the appreciation of the strengths in collaboration, and the greater the understanding of the increase in positive outcomes, on a case-by-case basis, attributable to the unique combined advanced skills of both professions.

FACTORS IN SUCCESSFUL COLLABORATION

If the interprofessional nurse–social worker team is seen as a small group, the dynamics of ongoing collaboration can be best understood and dealt with as the interaction evolves, and the usual stresses occur. Kane (1975) suggested that eight issues be considered in conceptualizing the collaborative team as a small group: the individual in the group; team size; group norms; democracy; decision making and conflict resolution; communication and structure; leadership; and group harmony and its relationship to group productivity.

The point is well taken that an individual professional's behavior on an interprofessional team is a product of group process as well as a function of frequently differing professional roles, statuses, investments, values, and skills. Thus, the collaborative team is a combination of both strengths and weaknesses and, as such, must be constantly and sensitively assessed in terms of its achievement of optimal combined outcomes of efficiency and effectiveness in the maintenance and promotion of health status.

CASE MANAGEMENT

Collaboration models are generated at the organizational, administrative, interorganizational, and community systems levels. Case management is the means by which collaborative systems models are operationalized at the individual and small systems levels (families and other small reference

COLLABORATION MODEL

(Organizational, Administrative, Interorganizational, and Community Levels)

↓   ↑

CASE MANAGEMENT

(Individual and Small Systems Levels—Families, Work Groups, and Peers)

FIGURE 5.1 Levels and interactions of collaboration models and case management.

groups such as work groups, and peers). Both levels are fluid and interact constantly, as Figure 5.1 shows.

Case management is the hot practice topic of the 1990s for both nursing and social work (Raiff & Shore, 1993). "Given the large demonstration of need, the growing cast of players, the pyramiding of research findings, and the lure of added dollars, it is little wonder that case management is now recognized as a core service" (Raiff & Shore, 1993, p. 7), variously termed, "perhaps the most essential unifying factor in service delivery" and "the energizing factor that has propelled the service plan into the reality of service delivery" (Behar, 1985, p. 194). In some settings, this function is termed "care management" (Berkman, et al., 1996). For purposes of this discussion, the more widely used and understood term "case management" will be employed.

The case management practice concept began in the early 1970s as an answer to burgeoning human services systems in the 1960s, which were "complex, fragmented, duplicative, uncoordinated, and inaccessible" (Raiff & Shore, 1993, p. 3). Since then a good deal has been written about this modality in a range of areas:

• General social work practice and the health, behavioral health, and human services (Austin, 1993; Johnson & Rubin, 1983; Kane, 1988; Kanter, 1992; Kisthardt & Rapp, 1992; Loomis, 1988; Moore, 1990; Moxley, 1989; National Association of Social Workers [NASW], 1992, 1995; Raiff & Shore, 1993; Roberts-DeGennaro, 1987; Rose, 1992a, 1992b; Rothman, 1991; Rubin, 1992; Seltzer, Ivry, & Litchfield, 1992; Weil, Karls, & Associates, 1988; Witheridge, 1992)
• Long-term care (Applebaum & Austin, 1990; Austin, 1983, 1993; Capitman, Haskins, & Bernstein, 1986; Collopy, 1992; Quinn, 1993)
• Geriatric practice (Azzarto, 1992; Downing, 1988)

- Children and child welfare (Wells, 1988)
- Developmentally disabled (Kailes & Weil, 1988)
- Physical disabilities (Kailes & Weil, 1988)
- Serious and chronic mental illness (Harris & Bergman, 1992; Honnard, 1988; Intagliata & Baker, 1983; Intagliata, 1992; Kanter, 1991; Libassi, 1992; Rife et al., 1991; Schwartz, Goldman, & Churgin, 1982; Surber, 1994).

The model of case management here assumes nurse–social worker collaboration as equal partners. The basic structure of the collaborative case management model will be outlined in this chapter. The operational components of the model will be described, with case examples, in chapter 6.

BIOPSYCHOSOCIAL INDIVIDUAL AND SYSTEMS INTERVENTION MODEL OF CASE MANAGEMENT IN THE COMMUNITY

The basic components of almost all case management systems are as follows:

1. Initial client outreach and engagement.
2. Assessment and diagnosis of needed services, programs, and resources.
3. Developing a service strategy (referred to as the plan of care or the service plan).
4. Linking clients to services and community resources identified in the plan (a crucial element is "priming" the system for ease of client access and linkage).
5. Implementation and coordination of effort to insure that programs are implemented in logical, stepwise fashion, and that they jointly address identified needs, which are pooled in the plan.
6. Monitoring and evaluation to determine the quality of fit between the client's state of being and current service deliverables.
7. Advocacy.
8. Preparing the client for termination of services (Raiff & Shore, 1993, p. 4).

Figure 5.2 depicts case management functions juxtaposed with meta variables in one recent conceptualization of a quality case management model (Raiff & Shore, 1993, p. 23). Case management is an umbrella practice concept, which encompasses specific functions (such as assess-

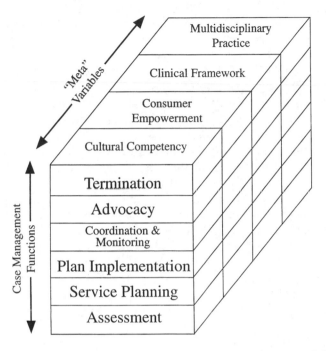

FIGURE 5.2   Matrix of quality care management practice: a model.

From N. R. Raiff with B. K. Shore (1993). *Advanced Case Management: New Strategies for the Nineties*, p. 23. Copyright © 1993 by Sage Publications. Reprinted by permission of Sage Publications, Inc.

ment, service planning, plan implementation, coordination and monitoring, advocacy, and termination), and so-called overarching meta variables (such as multidisciplinary practice, clinical framework, consumer empowerment, and cultural competency). Its breadth makes it a perfect framework for an interdisciplinary collaboration model.

Models of case management vary, from those that provide the bare minimum of services (outreach, assessment, planning, and referral), to more complex and sophisticated ones that offer advocacy, direct clinical work and casework, development of natural support systems, monitoring and evaluation of program outcomes, education for self-care (activities of daily living) or parenting, educating the community, crisis intervention, and medication management. Types of case management may be programmed to be episodic or available continuously throughout the life span.

Throughout its history, case management practice, in both nursing and social work, has faced the dilemma of whether its major stance is primarily for client advocacy or as a means for resource management and rationing. This conceptual confusion about the purposes of case management exists to this day, "co-mingling client-focused and cost-containment expectations and creating ongoing tension for staff and for the greater professional and lay communities" (Loomis, 1988, p. 224).

Rose (1992a, 1992b) pointed out that most case management systems are divided into those that are *provider driven* and those that are *client driven*. We prefer the term *client focused*, which is more in line with the interactive model being proposed here. Rose espoused the client-focused case management approach, one that stresses services delivery appropriate to clients' goals and needs; monitoring and assessing provider performance; and advocacy for and empowerment of clients, their families, and significant others. This model stresses empowerment, self-determination, autonomy, and client-centered focus on equal client participation in and choice about treatment and service plans.

Provider-driven case management, on the other hand, stresses cost containment, rationed care, coordination of care, efficiency, and accountability. Client input is minimal. The provider-driven view of case management

> presumes that the primary role of case manager derives from the treatment or service plans prepared by professional staff: responsibilities include providing linkage to the existing service delivery agencies; monitoring to assure patients' medication compliance and attendance at the activities specified by the provider's treatment plan; and providing transportation to assure concrete needs get attended. Advocacy applies only to case-by-case issues, restricted to such activities as assuring Medicaid eligibility. (Rose, 1992b, p. 73)

In the very common provider-driven framework for mental health case management, the appropriateness of services to clients' goals and needs is equated with the availability of services offered; assessing the effectiveness of services is reduced to measuring the efficiency of service delivery; the quality or outcome of services in clients' lives is equated with provider output or the quantity of services consumed; and the common failure to stabilize people in community settings is reduced to predictive diagnostic labels such as "treatment resistant" or "young adult chronic." (Rose, 1992b, p. 73)

Client-focused case management

in contrast, does not begin with treatment plans or service plans controlled by service providers or shaped by their funding formulas. It begins with a set of principles formulated to emphasize clients' potential; their dignity; their capacity to grow and develop when provided with adequate material resources (safe, affordable housing; income; jobs where appropriate; etc.); appropriate supports and assistance to focus on living stable, positive lives; and validation communicated through an ongoing commitment to empowerment. Clients' strengths, goals, or desired life directions take precedence over formal service provider resources as the point of orientation for case managers. (Rose, 1992b, p. 74)

These two underlying case management world views of "problem-defining frameworks" (Rose) need not be and should not be stark dichotomies. It is quite possible to combine these two seemingly polar stances in service delivery practice, and we propose to do so. The new model we propose must, of course, be tested in relation to its outcomes, as must much of current case management practice across human service groups and settings.

THE STRUCTURE OF THE BIOPSYCHOSOCIAL INDIVIDUAL AND SYSTEMS INTERVENTION MODEL OF NURSE–SOCIAL WORKER COLLABORATION

The proposed collaborative nurse–social worker case management service delivery model will have the following structural characteristics:

1. It is both client and system focused.
2. It provides advanced case management by advanced systems practitioners.
3. It uses clinical case management.
4. It provides a holistic view of the biopsychosocial person-in-situation (an excellent area to see nurse–social worker complementary approaches). For the nurse, holistic is the whole mind/body. For the social worker, holistic encompasses the entire ecosystem.
5. The BISIM has a life model, strengths, client competency enhancement conceptual framework.
6. The BISIM uses interdisciplinary team case management; the transdisciplinary model.
7. Roles will be differentiated between nurse and social worker on the team according to those tasks for which each is clearly best

trained and those tasks that may be undertaken by either one or both professions.

8. The BISIM is flexible in assessing community needs and responding to changes in individuals, groups, communities, and organizations.
9. It has a strong community health education and physical and mental illness prevention component.
10. The BISIM has a strong advocacy component.
11. It will be available as needed in the community throughout the life span.
12. The BISIM has a strong qualitative and quantitative monitoring and outcome evaluation accountability component.

The proposed model will be fleshed out conceptually here and discussed in its operational nurse–social worker collaborative form in the community in chapter 6.

CLIENT AND SYSTEM FOCUS

The National Association of Social Workers defines case management, as it is to be practiced by professional social workers, as "a method of providing services whereby a professional social worker assesses the needs of the client and the client's family, when appropriate, and arranges, coordinates, monitors, evaluates, and advocates for a package of multiple services to meet the specific client's complex needs" (*NASW*, 1992, p. 5). "The primary goal of case management is to optimize client functioning by providing quality services in the most efficient and effective manner to individuals with multiple complex needs" (*NASW*, 1992, p. 5). Although considerable variation may exist in terms of roles, responsibilities, tasks performed, and auspices of social work case management, the tasks performed are both client-level and system-level interventions. The BISIM being proposed here, therefore, combines individual and systems (family, group, community, and organizational) factors, and is both provider-driven (system) and client-driven (consumer) (Raiff & Shore, 1993; Rose, 1992a, 1992b).

ADVANCED CASE MANAGEMENT PROVIDED BY ADVANCED SYSTEMS PRACTITIONERS

Abramczyk (1989) pointed out that new case management programs have highly sophisticated assessment and intervention modes, and are much more ecologically (biopsychosocially) attuned; less wed to a strictly medical model of assessment, diagnosis, and treatment; and stress much more individual, family, group, and community strengths and competencies over harmful pathologies. Due to the breadth and depth of skills needed to successfully intervene as a case manager, and the autonomy, flexibility, and creativity to expand services' parameters and to evaluate services outcomes, the biopsychosocial model proposed here should be directed and supervised by nurses and social workers who, by both education and experience, are advanced level practitioners. In the home health care area, for example, social workers must have a master's degree, whereas nurses can have a bachelor's degree. Many of the line roles and tasks can be carried out by social workers with bachelor's degrees, registered nurses, paraprofessional staff, and, where appropriate, volunteer individuals and families.

The ubiquity and higher skill levels demanded by current and future human services case managers elevates and differentiates advanced case management from generalist practice and casework in social work (Raiff & Shore, 1993). Case management taken here is clearly an advanced practice specialty and, as such, must be performed by advanced systems practitioners.

CLINICAL CASE MANAGEMENT

The most controversial of advanced case management's aspects is that of clinical case manager. When service delivery veers from coordination and delivery of physical and environmental supports toward promoting intrapsychic client change, many advocates for the viability of the case management concept drop by the wayside.

Raiff and Shore described clinical case management as having

> a two-pronged thrust: it is more focused on the changes, options, and pacing of relationships than 'broker' models, and it weaves clinical understandings throughout the process of disposition planning, service referral, advocacy, and follow-up. Some view this as an advanced, more expert modality. It builds on an infrastructure of the generic skills of assessment, planning, linking, monitoring, and advocacy and weds this to client engagement, consultation, and collaboration to other treating clinicians, individual psychotherapy, psychoeducation, and crisis intervention. A clinically informed practice is manifested through the conduct of skilled biopsychosocial assessments, demonstrated understanding of different personality types and their needs, skill in tailoring the client's physical and social environment, and being able to intervene appropriately as the client's need for support and structure changes. (1993, pp. 85–86)

This level of clinical intervention requires senior nurses and social workers with considerable previous practice experience and backgrounds and training in psychopathology, interpersonal relationships, and group interventions at a variety of levels and with diverse populations.

HOLISTIC VIEW OF THE BIOPSYCHOSOCIAL PERSON-IN-SITUATION

Each situation will be viewed in its totality, meshing presenting and ongoing problems and issues with myriads of relevant factors important to problem resolution such as cultural, interactional, economic, family, culture, psychological, and social.

CONCEPTUAL FRAMEWORK: LIFE MODEL, STRENGTHS, COMPETENCY, ENHANCEMENT

The combined developmental models to be taken for practice include the Life Model of Germain and Gitterman (1980), the competence-oriented model of Maluccio (1981), and the strengths perspective model of Kisthardt and Rapp (1992) and Saleeby (1996). These will take precedence over traditional pathology models, sole emphasis on which has not proven particularly helpful for solving complex issues in community settings. The psychopathology model, with its reliance on rigid diagnostic and assessment categories (such as the American Psychiatric Association's (1994) *Diagnostic and statistical manual of mental disorders* (4th ed.) in the mental health area) and narrow-range explanations, has had very mixed outcome reviews, even when interventions using the model are confined to an in-office setting, serve middle-class clientele, and enjoy unlimited lengths of intervention time (in chapter 7 we will discuss diagnostic categories that are appropriate to the proposed biopsychosocial individual and systems intervention model).

INTERDISCIPLINARY TEAM CASE MANAGEMENT: A TRANSDISCIPLINARY MODEL

The relatively new transdisciplinary model borrowed from early education is recommended (McGonigel & Garland, 1988; Woodruff & McGonigel, 1987). It is suggested that this particular approach cuts down on many of the dysfunctional interdisciplinary collaboration issues mentioned previously, especially, "professionally fragmented, pluralistic theories of individual behavior and how to best meet needs" (Raiff & Shore, 1993, p. 90). The multidisciplinary team idea, an attempt to combine sometimes highly idiosyncratic approaches into a single, coherent service plan, has "become the 'gold standard' of quality care. Case managers are commonly assigned lead responsibility for initiating and coordinating multidisciplinary approaches for clients throughout all phases of the assessment-monitoring-evaluation cycle" (Raiff & Shore, from NASW, 1984, p. 90).

Problems with the traditional multidisciplinary team have been dealt with previously. For purposes of this discussion of the transdisciplinary model, a few important snags will be reiterated: inability to develop coherent service plans, chronic disagreement over diagnoses and assessments, and interminable arguments over diagnostic terminology and the reliability and viability of various testing procedures or observational acumen. Other trouble signs are rigidities of stances about plans, procedures, interventions, ritualism in service plan development, limited interdisciplinary respect, and other typical organizational dysfunction variables such as interprofessional blaming and name calling, and a harmful failure to share anything, be it language, perceptions, or values (Raiff & Shore, 1993, pp. 92–93). Two important things also frequently occur: client wishes and needs get lost, and team members become more isolated, bored, turned off, and burned-out.

The transdisciplinary model is perhaps the most promising interdisciplinary team model currently in operation. This model has

> encouraged widespread discussion of the volitional and situational nature of case management, role ownership, and how service delivery can be better coordinated using structured team learning and internal consultation as resource enhancement activities. This approach is associated with many innovations related to intake, assessment, and service planning. (Raiff & Shore, 1993, pp. 94–95)

Raiff and Shore (1993) pointed out that the two most important concepts in the transdisciplinary team model are *role release* and *consultation*. Role release represents the exchange of team member skills and information across disciplines toward increasing integration at the expense of fragmentation, one of the major potential problems in interdisciplinary team collaboration. In this model, team members learn terminology and the more basic interventions from each other, which expands the portability of team services. Consultation enables the constant learning within the team and more informed, from a variety of professional conceptual and skill perspectives, services delivery.

Operationally, the transdisciplinary model works as follows:

1. One person is designated to work directly with the consumer (cutting number of staff contacts and decreasing the need for consumers

to relate to numbers of professionals, which can cause confusion at best, and playing one or more team members against the other(s).
2. Within the team, all members are expected to constantly acquire new learning through internal consultation and supervision (Raiff & Shore, 1993, pp. 95–96).

An example of an early intervention outreach team, which employed the transdisciplinary team model, is shown in Table 5.1.

In all of its permutations, one thing is constant: the case manager's role is that of both practice specialist and team facilitator. This model, primarily because of its flexibility and services planning and delivery sophistication, is seen as difficult to instigate and administer because of staff time requirements for planning, service delivery, training, monitoring, and evaluation. However, its strengths in both client responsiveness and professional growth more than offset its administrative and organizational drawbacks.

ROLE DEFINITION ON TEAM BY TASKS

The specifics of role definition and differentiation will be discussed in chapter 6, "Finding Common Ground in the Community: Nurse and Social Worker Roles in Implementing the BISIM."

FLEXIBILITY IN ASSESSING COMMUNITY NEEDS AND RESPONDING TO CHANGES WITH CREATIVE SERVICES DELIVERY

This area will also be addressed in chapter 6.

STRONG COMMUNITY HEALTH EDUCATION AND PHYSICAL AND MENTAL ILLNESS PREVENTION COMPONENT

This area will also be addressed in chapter 6.

ADVOCACY COMPONENT

The advocacy component of professional intervention in the health and human services areas has, once again, come into high regard. In fact, a recent Aetna advertisement for its Informed Health Plan titled, "What's a Nurse Case Manager?," answers the question in part by asking another question: "Where can you find an advocate who will stick with you every step of the way, from diagnosis through recovery?" Both nursing and social work, as was pointed out in chapter 3, "Historical Origins," began

TABLE 5.1   Project Optimus: A Transdisciplinary Approach in Early Intervention Intake, Assessment, and Service Planning (Case Management with Children and Youth)

Project Optimus, an outreach program funded from 1978 to 1986 to provide transdisciplinary (TD) training in early intervention, developed a unique approach to assessment and service planning based on the position that responsibility could be rotated among team members. To avoid traditional labels, this lead person was referred to as the primary service provider (PSP). This project's TD approach used a multistage intake and assessment process, which included a preassessment intake and an elaborately prepared "arena assessment."

The intake was intended to engage the family, to acquire background data, and to provide the family with information about their partnership in the TD process. Intake information included previous use of services and diagnostic data. Other family-centered information collected was its view of the child's level of functioning, learning style, condition, and needs; data related to its support systems, stresses, and coping; behaviors; and the family's program expectations.

The intake helped family members to anticipate the arena and service options. Parents were encouraged to identify the best time for their child's assessment and to bring others to the assessment for moral support.

The team selected its roles prior to the arena assessment. An assessment facilitator was selected, and other team members provided consultation about appropriate developmental tools, areas of concern, and how to involve the family and child. The assessment facilitator was either the person who conducted the intake or another team member.

During the arena assessment, the facilitator worked with the child and parents. Other team members observed and recorded the child's behavior and the parent-child interactions. Parents had the option of being either participants or observers. They were encouraged to interpret their child's responses or to make suggestions about approaches that the facilitator might find useful.

The TD protocol called for postsession meetings for continued family input and debriefing, and for internal team development. The first session was conducted immediately after the arena assessment with the family and other team members. Here ideas were exchanged, the child's strengths and needs established, and the family's goals and priorities discussed.

A second postsession TD meeting was held for staff development and critique without the family present. Here the final PSP (case manager) assignment was made, and the team evaluated the assessment process. Finally, one team member, usually the PSP, developed a written report summarizing the team's findings and recommendations. This authorized the PSP to carry out the service plan with the family. All team members

(cont.)

TABLE 5.1 *(Continued)*

continued to provide the family and PSP with formal and informal support and backup services when complicated situations arose.

From: N. R. Raiff with B. K. Shore (1993). *Advanced Case Management: New Strategies for the Nineties*, p. 96. Copyright © 1993 by Sage Publications. Reprinted by permission of Sage Publications, Inc.

with strong advocacy components to their interventions on behalf of clients, groups, and communities. Indeed, almost everything undertaken by Jane Addams at Hull-House and Lillian Wald at the Henry Street Settlement had a strong advocacy thrust.

Both nursing and social work, in their mutual attempts to gain professional standing in medical institutions and social welfare bureaucracies, respectively, lost value for advocacy activities, considering them unprofessional generalist endeavors. Now that both professions have been thrust back into the community by managed care and, before that, by deinstitutionalization efforts, advocacy as a bona fide professional activity, one requiring advanced skills, is back in the ascendancy as an effective intervention mode.

Rose (1992a, 1992b) conceptualized an advocacy-empowerment design for case management activities, one that is predominantly client-focused rather than provider-driven. Rose provided a rationale for incorporating advocacy functions as an integral part of the team's services. He reminded us that social work cannot ''simply watch or rationalize oppression; benign or avid neglect for our roots are too closely tied to the client constituencies that have historically justified our existence. We need to generate new practice models, based on emerging practice paradigms to guide our way back to our roots'' (p. 296).

Available in the Community Throughout the Life Span

The model to be espoused is the continuous care team, a concept to be incorporated into the transdisciplinary team model described above. The continuous care team represents ''one of the more highly sophisticated, theoretically well-developed team case management models'' (Raiff & Shore, 1993, p. 133). The basic idea is that such teams are responsible for a given client constellation throughout the client's life span, continuously and indefinitely, regardless of the location of the client at any given point in time (for example, at home or with family in the community, or at a hospital, shelter, assisted living center, or residential placement). The transdisciplinary team takes responsibility for meeting client needs, both directly and indirectly, as these needs arise, thus providing clients and their families a consistent community-based health and behavioral health resource.

QUALITATIVE AND QUANTITATIVE MONITORING AND OUTCOME EVALUATION ACCOUNTABILITY COMPONENT

Program evaluation for decision making and accountability is essential in any service intervention, particularly one as complex and various as suggested for the BISIM (Honnard & Wolkon, 1988; McCarthy, Gelber, & Dugger, 1993). Agreement is strong that qualitative and quantitative monitoring and outcome evaluation must proceed at two major levels:

1. An assessment of the efficiency and effectiveness of both the collaborative process model itself and the broader policy, programmatic, and advocacy results of the application of the interdisciplinary collaborative model (Schlenker, Shaughnessy, & Crisler, 1995; Tweed & Weber, 1995). Few evaluations of interdisciplinary collaboration models have been implemented (Applebaum & Austin, 1990; Sowell & Meadows, 1994). The BISIM proposed should be evaluated in relation to both process and outcomes, using qualitative and quantitative measures, in whatever settings it is carried out. The evaluation process should be ongoing (Bartlett & Cohen, 1993) and should consist of measures agreed to and taken by all stakeholders in the collaborative team, professional case managers and other service deliverers, nonprofessionals, volunteers, administration, clients, and the communities served.

2. An assessment of the efficiency and effectiveness of case management service plans and delivery outcomes on clients and their families. Unlike the broader collaborative model area, several evaluations of case management services delivery models have been undertaken (Chamberlain & Rapp, 1991; Korr & Cloninger, 1991; Rothman, 1991; Thompson, Burns, Goldman, & Smith, 1992). The task of outcome evaluation, mandated by managed care systems, needs to be addressed in ongoing fashion by any interdisciplinary team. There are three major components of outcome evaluations: protocol development and initial goal setting; measuring outcomes reliably and validly; and effectively utilizing outcome data for programmatic change, policy implementation, and individuals and systems advocacy.

Protocol Development and Initial Goal Setting

Nursing has developed protocols (frequently termed care pathways or critical pathways) for almost every nursing care area (examples are Beyea,

1996 and Hawkins et al., 1997). Social work is attempting to generate protocols, especially in the home health care sector, to "identify social and emotional problems impacting the patient's medical condition, treatment plan, or rate of recovery together with the establishment of a social work treatment plan and clear and concise documentation of findings" (Williams, 1995; see also Williams, 1991).

The need to define both initial and ongoing goals to cast outcomes against them at some outcome point is essential. Ashley pointed out the pitfalls of the interdisciplinary team not clearly articulating initial goals this way, "if the objective of case management services is not well defined and articulated, it is likely that conflicts will escalate and everyone will end up dissatisfied with the outcome" (1988, p. 499). Further, once a goal is agreed on, other decisions, such as what professional qualifications and experience the case manager in a particular situation should have, will be easier to answer, in addition to being crucial to outcome assessments (Ashley, 1988).

The interdisciplinary team that agrees on the initial goals should build evaluation into its group ethos; develop ways to share the burden of data collection and analysis; and simplify data input and analysis by use of computer technology to classify, codify, analyze, and interpret. The strength of having the entire interdisciplinary team engage in the outcome evaluation process from initial protocol and goal setting through data analysis, in a sense to own it, has been noted by several observers (Kiser, Heston, Millsap, & Pruitt, 1991; Stichler, 1995).

Measuring Outcomes Reliably and Validly

The interdisciplinary team should agree on existing outcome measures or should design its own. The most sensitive means of measuring (a) whether improvements are due to the interventions or to other actors and factors; (b) in whose opinion (clients, families, professionals, managed care companies) has improvement occurred; and (c) what are viable outcome measures are all matters of controversy. The outcome measures will be improved if clients are involved from the initial assessment and goal-setting stages through outcome and follow-up assessments. That the proposed model posits a womb-to-tomb connection with clients and their families and significant others affords multiple opportunities for measurement by the interdisciplinary team.

Case recording methods are important for quality assurance reviews, ongoing monitoring, and outcome evaluations (Corcoran & Gingerich, 1994). The Goal Attainment Scaling data measurement model developed by Kiresuk, Smith, and Cardillo (1994) offers a parsimonious, yet reliable and valid, outcome measurement technique. Numerous other measurement tools have been employed, particularly in the area of clinical practice in social work (Benbenishty, 1988; Benbenishty, Ben-Zaken, & Yekel, 1991; Flowers & Booarem, 1990; Thompson, 1985; Zinober, Dinkel, & Windle, 1984).

Effectively Utilizing Outcome Data for Programmatic Change, Policy Implementation, and Individuals and Systems Advocacy

Because nurses and social workers see themselves both as uniquely trained and skilled in methods of collaboration, particularly its communication aspects, and in case management, the settings in which the two professions interact are fertile for misunderstanding, competition, and lack of cooperative pooling of different talents (sometimes because these are not seen as different at all). How this can be worked out operationally by applying the BISIM will be seen in chapter 6.

REFERENCES

Abramczyk, L. W. (1989). *Social work education for working with seriously emotionally disturbed children and adolescents.* Paper presented at a symposium on social work education and child mental health, sponsored by the National Association of Deans and Directors of Schools of Social Work (NADDSSW). Charleston, SC: National Association of Deans and Directors of Schools of Social Work.

Abramson, J. S., & Mizrahi, T. (1996a). Strategies for enhancing collaboration between social workers and physicians. *Social Work in Health Care, 12,* 1–21.

Abramson, J. S., & Mizrahi, T. (1996b). When social workers and physicians collaborate: Positive and negative interdisciplinary experiences. *Social Work, 41,* 270–281.

Abramson, J. S., & Rosenthal, B. B. (1995). Interdisciplinary and interorganizational collaboration. *Encyclopedia of Social Work* (19th ed., Vol. II, pp. 1479–1489).

Andrews, A. B. (1987). Interdisciplinary and interorganizational collaboration. *Encyclopedia of Social Work* (18th ed. [Suppl.], pp. 175–188). Silver Spring, MD: National Association of Social Workers. (Ed-in-Chief: Anne Minahan.)

Applebaum, R., & Austin, C. (1990). *Long-term care case management: Design and evaluation.* New York: Springer.

Ashley, A. (1988). Case management: The need to define goals. *Hospital and Community Psychiatry, 39*(5), 499–500.

Austin, C. D. (1983). Case management in long-term care: Options and opportunities. *Health and Social Work,* 16–30.

Austin, C. D. (1993). Case management: A systems perspective. *Families in Society,* 451–459.

Azzarto, J. (1992). Medicalization of the problems of the elderly. In S. M. Rose (Ed.), *Case management and social work practice* (pp. 189–198). White Plains, NY: Longman.

Bartlett, J., & Cohen, J. (1993). Building an accountable, improvable delivery system. *Administration and Policy in Mental Health, 21*(1), 51–58.

Behar, L. (1985). Changing patterns of state responsibility: A case study of North Carolina. *Journal of Clinical Child Psychology, 14*, 188–195.

Benbenishty, R. (1988). Assessment of task-centered interventions with families in Israel. *Journal of Social Service Research, 11*(4), 19–43.

Benbenishty, R., Ben-Zaken, A., & Yekel, H. (1991). Monitoring interventions with young Israeli families. *British Journal of Social Work, 21*, 143–155.

Berger, C. S., Cayner, J., Jensen, G., Mizrahi, T., Scesny, A., & Trachtenberg, J. (1996, August). The changing scene of social work in hospitals: A report of a national study by the Society for Social Work Administrators in Health Care and NASW. *Health and Social Work, 21*(3), 167–177.

Berkman, B., Shearer, S., Simmons, W. J., White, M., Robinson, M., Sampson, S., Holmes, W., Allison, D., & Thomson, J. A. (1996). Ambulatory elderly patients of primary care physicians: Functional, psychosocial and environmental predictors of need for social work care management. *Social Work in Health Care, 22*(3), 1–20.

Beyea, S. C. (1996). *Critical pathways for collaborative nursing care.* Menlo Park, CA: Addison-Wesley.

Capitman, J. A., Haskins, B., & Bernstein, J. (1986). Case management approaches in coordinated community-oriented long-term care demonstrations. *Gerontologist, 26*, 398–404.

Carlton, T. O. (1984). *Clinical social work in health settings. A guide to professional practice with exemplars.* New York: Springer.

Chamberlain, R., & Rapp, C. A. (1991). A decade of case management: A methodological review of outcome research. *Community Mental Health Journal, 37*, 171–188.

Collopy, B. (1992). Autonomy in long-term care. Some future directions. In S. M. Rose (Ed.), *Case management and social work practice* (pp. 56–71). White Plains, NY: Longman.

Corcoran, K., & Gingerich, W. J. (1994). Practice evaluation in the context of managed care: Case recording methods for quality assurance reviews. *Research on Social Work Practice, 4*, 326–337.

Cowles, L. A., & Lefcowitz, M. J. (1992). Interdisciplinary expectations of the medical social worker in the hospital setting. *Health and Social Work, 17*, 57–65.

Dane, B. O., & Simon, B. L. (1991). Resident guests: Social workers in host settings. *Social Work, 36*, 208–213.

Downing, R. (1988). The elderly and their families. In M. Weil & J. M. Karls (Eds.), *Case management in human service practice* (pp. 145–169). San Francisco: Jossey-Bass.

Encyclopedia of Social Work (1987). 18th ed. Silver Spring, MD: National Association of Social Workers. (Ed-in-Chief: Anne Minahan.)

Encyclopedia of Social Work (1995). 19th ed. Washington, DC: National Association of Social Workers. (Ed-in-Chief: Richard L. Edwards.)

Flowers, J. V., & Booarem, C. D. (1990). Four studies toward an empirical foundation for group therapy. *Advances in Group Work Research*, 105–121.

Frangos, A. S., & Chase, D. (1976). Potential partners: Attitudes of family practice residents toward collaboration with social workers in their future practices. *Social Work in Health Care, 2*(1), 65–76.

Germain, C. B., & Gitterman, A. (1980). *The life model of social work practice.* New York: Columbia University Press.

Harris, M., & Bergman, H. C. (1992). Case management with the chronically mentally ill. A clinical perspective. In S. M. Rose (Ed.), *Case management and social work practice* (pp. 91–100). White Plains, NY: Longman.

Hawkins, J. W., Roberto, D. M., & Stanley-Haney, J. L. (1997). *Protocols for nurse practitioners in gynecological settings.* New York: Tiresias.

Honnard, R. (1988). The chronically mentally ill in the community. In M. Weil & J. M. Karls (Eds.), *Case management in human service practice* (pp. 204–232). San Francisco: Jossey-Bass.

Honnard, R., & Wolkon, G. H. (1988). Evaluation for decision making and program accountability. In M. Weil & J. M. Karls (Eds.), *Case management in human service practice* (pp. 94–118). San Francisco: Jossey-Bass.

Intagliata, J. (1992). Improving the quality of community care for the chronically mentally disabled: The role of case management. In S. M. Rose (Ed.), *Case management and social work practice* (pp. 25–55). White Plains, NY: Longman.

Intagliata, J., & Baker, F. (1983). Factors affecting case management services for the chronically mentally ill. *Administration in Mental Health, 11*(2), 75–91.

Johnson, P. J., & Rubin, A. (1983). Case management in mental health: A social work domain? *Social Work, 28*, 49–55.

Kailes, J. I., & Weil, M. (Eds.). (1988). People with physical disabilities and the independent living model. In M. Weil & J. M. Karls, *Case management in human service practice* (pp. 276–316). San Francisco: Jossey-Bass.

Kane, R. A. (1975). The interprofessional team as a small group. *Social Work in Health Care, 1*, 19–32.

Kane, R. A. (1988). Case management in health care settings. In M. Weil & J. M. Karls, *Case management in human service practice* (pp. 170–203). San Francisco: Jossey-Bass.

Kanter J. S. (1991). Integrating case management and psychiatric hospitalization. *Health and Social Work, 16*, 34–42.

Kanter, J. S. (1992). Mental health case management. A professional domain? In S. M. Rose (Ed.), *Case management and social work practice* (pp. 126–130). White Plains, NY: Longman.

Kiresuk, T. J., Smith, A., & Cardillo, J. E. (Eds.). (1994). *Goal attainment scaling: Applications, theory, and measurement.* Hillsdale, NJ: Lawrence Erlbaum Associates.

Kiser, L. J., Heston, J. D., Millsap, P. A., & Pruitt, D. B. (1991). Treatment protocols in child and adolescent day treatment. *Hospital and Community Psychiatry, 42*(6), 597–600.

Kisthardt, W. E., & Rapp, C. A. (1992). Bridging the gap between principles and practice. Implementing a strengths perspective in case management. In S. M. Rose (Ed.), *Case management and social work practice* (pp. 112–125). White Plains, NY: Longman.

Koeske, G. F., Koeske, R. D., & Mallinger, J. (1993). Perceptions of professional competence: Cross-disciplinary ratings of psychologists, social workers, and psychiatrists. *American Journal of Orthopsychiatry, 63*, 45–54.

Korr, W. S., & Cloninger, L. (1991). Assessing models of case management: An empirical approach. *Journal of Social Service Research, 14*(1/2), 129–146.

Kulys, R., & Davis, M. A. Sr. (1987). Nurses and social workers: Rivals in the provision of social services? *Health and Social Work*, *12*, 101–111.

Lee, S. (1980). Interdisciplinary teaming in primary care: A process of evolution and revolution. *Social Work in Health Care*, *5*, 237–244.

Libassi, M. F. (1992). The chronically mentally ill. A practice approach. In S. M. Rose (Ed.), *Case management and social work practice* (pp. 77–90). White Plains, NY: Longman.

Loomis, J. F. (1988). Case management in health care. *Health and Social Work*, *13*, 219–225.

Lowe, J. I., & Herranan, M. (1978). Conflict in teamwork: Understanding roles and relationships. *Social Work in Health Care*, *3*, 323–330.

Lowe, J. I., & Herranan, M. (1981). Understanding teamwork: Another look at the concepts. *Social Work in Health Care*, *7*(2), 1–11.

Maluccio, A. N. (Ed.). (1981). *Promoting competence in clients. A new/old approach to social work practice*. New York: Free Press.

McCarthy, P. R., Gelber, S., & Dugger, D. E. (1993). Outcome measurement to outcome management: The critical step. *Administration and Policy in Mental Health*, *21*, 59–68.

McGonigel, M. J., & Garland, C. (1988). The individualized family service plan and the early intervention plan: Team and family issues and recommended practices. *Infants and Young Children*, *1*, 10–21.

Mizrahi, T., & Abramson, J. (1985). Sources of strain between physicians and social workers: Implications for social workers in health care settings. *Social Work in Health Care*, *10*(3), 33–51.

Moore, S. T. (1990). A social work practice model of case management: The case management grid. *Social Work*, *35*(5), 444–448.

Moxley, D. P. (1989). *The practice of case management*. Newbury Park, CA: Sage.

National Association of Social Workers. (1984). *NASW standards and guidelines for social work case management for the functionally impaired* (Professional Standards, Number 12). Washington, DC: NASW Press.

National Association of Social Workers standards for social work case management. (1992, June). National Association of Social Workers: Case Management Standards Work Group, Washington, DC: NASW Press.

National Association of Social Workers clinical indicators for social work and psychosocial services in home health care. (1995, June). Washington, DC: NASW Press.

Netting, F. E., & Williams, F. G. (1996). Case manager-physician collaboration: Implications for professional identity, roles, and relationships. *Health and Social Work*, *21*(3), 216–224.

Quinn, J. (1993). *Successful case management in long-term care*. New York: Springer.

Raiff, N. R. (with Shore, B. K.) (1993). *Advanced case management. New strategies for the nineties*. Newbury Park, CA: Sage.

Rawlins, R. P., & Heacock, P. E. (1993). *Clinical manual of psychiatric nursing*. St. Louis, MO: Mosby.

Rife, J. C., First, R. J., Greenlee, R. W., Miller, L. D., & Feichter, M. A. (1991). Case management with homeless mentally ill people. *Health and Social Work*, *16*, 58–67.

Roberts, C. S. (1989). Conflicting professional values in social work and medicine. *Health and Social Work*, 211–218.

Roberts-DeGennaro, M. (1987). Developing case management as a practice model. *Social Casework, 68*, 466–470.

Rose, S. M. (Ed.). (1992a). Case management. An advocacy/empowerment design. In S. M. Rose, *Case management and social work practice* (pp. 271–297). White Plains, NY: Longman.

Rose, S. M. (1992b). *Case management and social work practice.* White Plains, NY: Longman.

Rothman, J. (1991). A model of case management: Toward empirically based practice. *Social Work, 36*(6), 520–528.

Rubin, A. (1992). Case management. In S. M. Rose (Ed.), *Case management and social work practice* (pp. 5–20). White Plains, NY: Longman.

Saleeby, D. (1992). *The strengths perspective in social work practice.* White Plains, NY: Longman.

Saleeby, D. (1996). The strengths perspective in social work practice: Extensions and cautions. *Social Work, 41*, 296–305.

Saltz, C. C., & Schaefer, T. (1996). Interdisciplinary teams in health care: Integration of family caregivers. *Social Work in Health Care, 22*(3), 59–70.

Sands, R. G. (1989). The social worker joins the team: A look at the socialization process. *Social Work, 34*(2), 1–14.

Sands, R. G., Stafford, J., & Mc Clelland, M. (1990). 'I beg to differ': Conflict in the interdisciplinary team. *Social Work in Health Care, 14*(3), 55–72.

Schlenker, R. E., Shaughnessy, P. W., & Crisler, K. S. (1995). Outcome-based continuous quality improvement as a financial strategy for home health care agencies. *Journal of Home Health Care Practice, 7*(4), 1–15.

Schwartz, S. R., Goldman, H. H., & Churgin, S. (1982). Case management for the chronically mentally ill: Models and dimensions. *Hospital and Community Psychiatry, 33*, 1006–1009.

Seltzer, M. M., Ivry, J., & Litchfield, L. C. (1992). Family members as case managers. Partnership between the formal and informal support networks. In S. M. Rose (Ed.), *Case management and social work practice* (pp. 229–242). White Plains, NY: Longman.

Sheppard, M. (1992). Contact and collaboration with general practitioners: A comparison of social workers and community psychiatric nurses. *British Journal of Social Work, 22*, 419–436.

Sowell, R. L., & Meadows, T. M. (1994). An integrated case management model: Developing standards, evaluation, and outcome criteria. *Nursing Administration Quarterly, 18*(2), 53–64.

Stichler, J. F. (1995). Professional interdependence: The art of collaboration. *Advanced Practice Nursing Quarterly, 1*, 53–61.

Surber, R. W. (Ed.). (1994). *Clinical case management. A guide to comprehensive treatment of serious mental illness.* Thousand Oaks, CA: Sage.

Thompson, C. M. (1985). Characteristics associated with outcome in a community mental health partial hospitalization program. *Community Mental Health Journal, 21*(3), 179–188.

Thompson, J. W., Burns, B. J., Goldman, H. H., & Smith, J. (1992). Initial level of care and clinical status in a managed mental health program. *Hospital and Community Psychiatry, 43*(6), 599–603.

Tweed. S. C., & Weber, A. J. (1995). Critical measures of success: A tool for organizational effectiveness, communication, and continuous improvement in home health care. *Journal of Home Health Care Practice*, 7(4), 64–68.

Weil, M., & Karls, J. M., & Associates (1988). *Case management in human service practice*. San Francisco, CA: Jossey-Bass.

Wells, S. J. (1988). Children and the child welfare system. In M. Weil & J. M. Karls (Eds.), *Case management inhuman service practice* (pp. 119–144). San Francisco, CA: Jossey-Bass.

Williams, E. K. (1991). *Guidelines and documentation requirements for social workers in home health care*. Unpublished manuscript.

Williams, E. K. (1995). Understanding social work in the home health care setting. *Journal of Home Health Care Practice*, 7(2), 12–20.

Witheridge, T. F. (1992). The assertive community treatment worker. An emerging role and its implications for professional training. In S. M. Rose (Ed.), *Case management and social work practice* (pp. 101–111). White Plains, NY: Longman.

Woodruff, G., & McGonigel, M. J. (1987). Early intervention team approaches: The transdisciplinary model. In J. Jordan, J. Gallagher, P. Huntinger, & M. Karns (Eds.), *Early childhood special education: Birth to three* (pp. 163–182). Reston, VA: Council for Exceptional Children.

Zinober, J. W., Dinkel, N. R., & Windle, C. (1984). Nonspecialist evaluation of mental health agencies. *Administration in Mental Health*, 11(4), 223–232.

CHAPTER 6

Finding Common Ground in the Community: Nurse and Social Worker Roles in Implementing the BISIM

Susan L. Williams and Nancy W. Veeder

Nurses and social workers on the interdisciplinary collaborative team must operationalize the Biopsychosocial Individual and Systems Intervention Model (BISIM) and carry out, in coordinated and comprehensive fashion, the roles, tasks, and functions that make up the BISIM service delivery package. In this chapter, an overview of nurse and social worker roles will be described, including similarities and differences, as well as specific examples of nurses and social workers working together on individual cases and with families in the community. The community auspices in the examples are home health care settings. Home health care settings were selected to exemplify nurse–social worker collaborative efforts in the community because home health care is one of the most rapidly expanding services delivery settings in the community for both health and behavioral health care, from prevention, through ameliorative, to tertiary and terminal care needs.

THE BISIM REVISITED

The characteristics of the proposed BISIM (described conceptually in chapter 5) determine roles, tasks, and functions to be carried out and coordinated into a seamless nurse–social worker collaborative team services delivery package. These characteristics are (a) client and system focus; (b) provision of advanced case management by advanced systems practitioners; (c) clinical case management focus; (d) provision of a holistic view of the biopsychosocial person-in-situation; (e) a life-model, strengths, client competency enhancement conceptual framework; (f) a transdisciplinary model of team case management; (g) differentiation between nurse and social worker functions on the basis of those tasks for which each is clearly best trained and those tasks that may be undertaken by either one or both professions; (h) flexibility in assessing community needs and responding to changes in individuals, groups, communities, and organizations; (i) a strong community health education and physical and mental illness prevention component; (j) a strong advocacy component; (k) availability in the community as needed throughout the life span; and (l) a strong qualitative and quantitative monitoring and outcome evaluation accountability component.

TASKS, ROLES, PERCEPTIONS OF NURSES AND SOCIAL WORKERS: WHAT IS THE PROPER "FIT"?

Table 6.1 depicts the direct and indirect tasks that must be performed in any case management effort, regardless of the profession carrying out these tasks.

The number of case management functions is vast. The interventions are complex. The possibilities for disagreement about who should do what are numerous.

The National Association of Social Workers (NASW) rightly points out that, "it is the control over the flow of clients, information, services, and funding that empowers the case manager and promotes his or her effectiveness in enhancing system functioning" (National Association of Social Workers (NASW), 1992, p. 118). NASW emphasizes that all of this is related to the degree of formal authority vested in the case manager role. Social work and nursing both have had difficulty with the vesting of authority by other professions and the bureaucracies and systems within which they have traditionally operated. Another problem has been sorting out which profession should have authority to perform which functions.

Kulys and Davis (1987, pp. 103, 107), studying nurse and social worker perceptions of who was most qualified to perform tasks in a hospice setting, found the following:

1. Assessment of physical problems (social workers: both social worker and nurse; nurses: nurse).

TABLE 6.1   Comprehensive Community-Based Team Case Management Tasks (Direct and Indirect Tasks)

Individual case-based case management

Direct services (individuals focused)

1. short-term therapy; crisis intervention and stabilization; education
2. assistance with daily living activities
3. financial counseling
4. cultural brokers
5. case identification/finding and outreach
6. psychosocial assessment
7. service planning
8. follow-up
9. mediation
10. case management

Indirect services (systems focused)

1. services linkage
2. services coordination
3. advocacy
4. monitoring services delivery
5. problem identification
6. team collaboration
7. networking
8. outreach
9. assessment
10. care planning
11. implementation
12. monitoring services delivery/quality assurance
13. reassessment
14. team collaboration
15. case conferencing
16. program development
17. outcome evaluation

Community-based systems case management

1. coordination of services
2. resource development
3. social action
4. agency policy formation

(cont.)

TABLE 6.1 *(Continued)*

5. data collection
6. information management
7. program evaluation
8. quality assurance
9. referral brokers
10. service management—responsible for costs of care plans developed
11. systems analysis
12. strategy development
13. identify and document service delivery effects, barriers, and obstacles originating at the system level
14. document the impact of newly implemented policies
15. policy development
16. research

Adapted, in part, from National Association of Social Workers (1992). *Standards of Social Work Case Management*. Annapolis Junction, MD: NASW Press.

2. Assessment of emotional and social problems (social workers: both social worker and nurse; nurses: social worker).
3. Evaluation of functional abilities (social workers: social worker; nurses: nurse).
4. Provision of information to other facilities (social workers: social worker; nurses: social worker).
5. Coordination of services (social workers: social worker; nurses: both social worker and nurse).
6. Provision of help to patients with emotional problems (social workers: social worker; nurses: nurse).
7. Provision of help to families with emotional problems (social workers: social worker [100%]; nurses: nurse [67%]).
8. Continuation of contact when death is imminent (social workers: social worker; nurses: nurse).
9. Discharge planning (social workers and nurses: both social worker and nurse).
10. Inducement of feelings of hope and acceptance (social workers: social worker; nurses: nurse).
11. Discussion of terminal illness with families (social workers: social worker; nurses: nurse).
12. Communication of patients' needs to team (social workers: social worker; nurses: nurse).
13. Documentation of discharge summaries (social workers: nurse; nurses: nurse).

14. Telephoning of clergy (social workers: social worker; nurses: nurse).

The only agreement between nurses and social workers was on assessment of physical problems, assessment of emotional and social problems, discharge planning, and documentation of discharge summaries. Conclusions in this study were that nurses in this sample viewed the performance of social services as part of their responsibility. For example, nurses saw the provision of psychosocial support, an area traditionally claimed by social work, as their domain, particularly in relation to support to individuals with emotional problems (67% of nurses thought nurses should perform this task) and support to families with emotional problems (67% of nurses also thought they did this best). Nurses (78%) also thought that they performed the task of inducing feelings of hope and acceptance best. Most practicing social workers would disagree with this perception on the part of nurses in the sample.

Figure 6.1 shows a basic model of nurse–social work collaboration in the community. Essentially, the biosocial nursing system is combined with the psychosocial social work system into the biopsychosocial model, which, in turn, informs collaborative case management efforts in the community. On a case-by-case basis, nursing and social work intervention

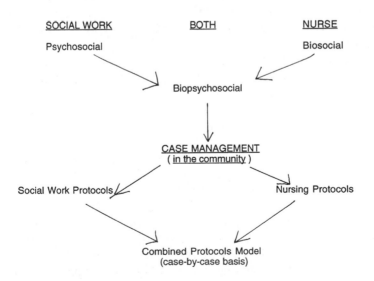

FIGURE 6.1 Model of nurse–social work collaboration in the community.

and treatment protocols are combined, or separated, according to client need and professional training. This will be discussed in the next section.

PUTTING THE TEAM TOGETHER IN THE COMMUNITY: HOME HEALTH CARE AS THE LABORATORY

The home health care arena provides an ideal environment in which to explore the boundaries and the content of collaborative nurse and social work roles. Both professions are charged with the mission of maximizing the client's ability to cope with illness and disability. The overriding goal is client compliance with the medical regimen or protocols. The same barriers to improved healing may be represented in both the nursing and social work treatment plans, or protocols. However, identified problems such as sleep disturbances, undernutrition, and medical noncompliance, are assessed and treated from two very different professional spheres of the nursing and social work domains. Although the two treatment plans may overlap, the core area of work is discipline specific and not interchangeable.

Table 6.2 depicts differences in nurse and social work domains and approaches.

Nursing education and training focus first on the physical sphere of a person, with subsequent integration of psychosocial considerations. Social work education and training concentrate first on the psychosocial sphere of the individual or system, with secondary attention being given to physical factors.

Some critical areas help define core differences between nursing and social work. For example, nursing role expectations and training necessitate access to a person's body, the infliction of pain and discomfort, and a micro view of the individual and organ systems. A skilled nurse learns how to cross the physical boundaries of a person with respect, providing as much comfort as is possible, depending on the procedure. Medical language such as "patient" and "noncompliance" reflect clearly that the locus of control is with the health care provider.

In sharp contrast to the nursing focus on the physical body, a social worker primarily attends to a client's psychological, social, and cultural boundaries and defenses. A successful social work connection and relationship depends on the client's ability and willingness to lower his or her emotional defenses. Social work assessments and interventions necessitate a macro focus of the person-in-the-environment, frequently called the individual's ecosystem. Unlike the primarily individual focus of the nurse,

TABLE 6.2   Differences in Nurse and Social Worker Domains

Nurse (Physical sphere)		Social Worker (Psychic sphere)
1. "Patient"/"client"	"Consumer"	1. "Client"
2. Access to body/mind		2. Access to emotions
3. Inflict physical pain		3. Open psychic pain
4. Touch body anywhere (including genitals)		4. Absolute touching taboo (except superficial touch with permission of client)
5. Soft boundaries re: confidentiality (among caregiving team members)		5. Hard boundaries re: confidentiality
6. Micro focus—organ systems; focus on individual		6. Macro focus—person-in-the-environment; group dynamics
7. Education in physical and psychosocial sphere, e. g., interpretation of "body language" as primarily physical		7. Education in psychosocial sphere, e. g., a different "lens" for "body language"
8. Locus of control: health care provider		8. Locus of control: client
Middle meeting ground (collaborative combining of domains) = biopsychosocial sphere		

social workers work from a systemic perspective with the client, not the medical system and its providers, holding the locus of control.

A major strength of the combined nurse–social worker collaborative team is that the total person is served. The best of both worlds is achieved because the client has the comfort and safety of maintaining defenses [in the psychological sphere with the nurse and in the physical sphere with the social worker]. For example, the nurse who gives an enema cannot be expected to finish that task and immediately take on the exploration of a client's feelings about being in a dangerous emotional or physical abuse situation. In the feelings-about-abuse situation, the client needs the comfort and safety of maintaining defenses in the physical sphere to be freed up in the emotional sphere. The separation of these two human spheres into clear roles and tasks from the client's perspective is what makes the serving of the total person by the two professions so necessary and so powerful.

The two professions differ, too, in terms of availability of protocols and practice guidelines. In home health, the nursing role entails a core list of concrete goals and corresponding tasks. Concise protocols and practice guidelines exist for most if not all nursing interventions. The social work role, on the other hand, is less clearly defined and frequently not guided by concise protocols.

Articulation of the social work role presents challenges even to advanced-level social work practitioners. Some of the most difficult (and potent) components of social work practice are either not articulated, or they are described in nonanalytic and non-intervention-prescriptive soft, passive, and mushy terms such as "supported and counseled the client." Nonetheless, home health social workers are frequently required to engage and establish a therapeutic environment with a defended and reluctant client and family, all within a complex home setting. The outcome of the medical treatment plan may depend almost totally on the social worker's ability to align with the clients and assist them in accepting, owning, and following through on treatment plans that support maximum health. Advanced skills are clearly required to experience success in engaging clients in mutual planning under these circumstances.

Most of the frequently stated social work interventions, such as psychosocial assessment, community resource planning, and crisis intervention, depend on the rarely stated task of client engagement. This crucial task needs to be operationalized and concretized with tasks. Because teamwork is enhanced by role clarification, social work has work to do in the area of professional role definition and interventions protocols development.

CASE EXAMPLES OF COLLABORATION

Two examples will be described to support previous conceptual discussions. Both composite cases from a home health care setting are presented with nurse and social work discipline-specific treatment plans and joint plans to demonstrate both the separate and collaborative work within the nurse–social work team.

CASE 1: MRS. WHITE

Mrs. White is an elderly woman who lives alone in her geographically isolated home (see Figure 6.2; Case 1, Medical Social Services Referral). Mrs. White was referred because she "lives alone, has minimal supports, husband died 3 years ago, congestive heart failure, increased episodes of

Patient: Rose White   DOB: _____   ID#: _____

Primary Care Physician _____ Other M.D. _____ SOP: _____

Disciplines Involved: ☑ VN ❐ HHA ❐ PT ❐ OT ❐ ST Contact in home: Pt or: ____

REASON FOR REFERRAL (check all that apply): ☑ High Priority

☑ Psychosocial assessment ❐ Health Care Proxy ❐ Arrange for alternate living situation

☑ Community resource planning ❐ Caregiver stress ☑ Frequent hospital visits or contacts

❐ Life style change due to disease ☑ Depression ❐ QD or BID VN visits

☑ Medication/Tx noncompliance ☑ Grief ❐ Abuse/neglect or domestic violence indicators

❐ Marital/family relationships ❐ Finances

☑ Safety/environmental issues ❐ Substance abuse

Other: Lives alone, minimal supports, husband died three years ago, CHF, increased episodes of angina, weight loss, med. non-compliance, refuses HHA.

Referred by: Hospital Social Worker Date: ____ Projected duration of VN Service: ____
MSS Form 1 4/96   Medication Profile and Nursing Narratives are attached.

FIGURE 6.2   Case 1 medical social services referral.

From: Visiting Nurse & Health Services. A program of Franklin Medical Center, Greenfield, MA. A member of Baystate Health Systems.

---

angina, weight loss, medication noncompliance, refuses home health aide.'' Several team interventions were requested. Among them were psychosocial assessment and community resource planning with the goal of medication-treatment compliance, safety-environmental issues, depression, grief, and frequent hospital visits or contacts. The social work intake was completed within 24 hours of referral due to the high priority status of the case.

The social worker, Jan, found Mrs. White to be depressed and initially very defended. Jan explained her role and pointed out that Mrs. White's sadness relative to her illness and significant losses was normal. As the social worker began to engage Mrs. White, she became less defended. Jan's careful and respectful questioning revealed the trigger for her recent medical and emotional decompensation. Her husband of 51 years had died 3 years ago that month. She expressed the desire to join her husband. She described

NAME: Rose White   DATE: 6/29/96

Problems or concerns:

Feels sad and hopeless - Anniversary date of husband's death three years ago.
Evenings especially difficult.

Plan:

   1. Increase home services for two weeks.
       • Social worker twice a week - Monday & Friday
       • HHA daily - late afternoon.
       • Increase Nursing visits to weekly.
   2. Sunday PM Support calls from elder cousin.
   3. Evening rituals - listen to music with dog near by.
   4. Call Emergency Services anytime day or night if support is needed (number
      near phone)

Client: _____

Social Worker: _____

Original to Patient   Yellow to MSS Chart

For CRISIS PREVENTION copies of WORK PLAN go to:
   • Primary Nurse
   • Nurse Manger
   • Evening, Night and Weekend Nurses
   • HHA Department

FIGURE 6.3   Case 1 medical social services work plan.

From: Visiting Nurse & Health Services. A program of Franklin Medical Center, Greenfield, MA.
A member of Baystate Health Systems.

a decrease in appetite, poor sleep, and a general disinterest in life in the
past month. She was assessed to be a level I suicide risk according to the
Suicide Risk Assessment protocol. Jan offered psychoeducation regarding
the power of anniversary dates on our mental and physical health.

Together they made a safety-self-nurturing plan (see Figure 6.3-Case
1, *Medical Social Services Work Plan*). The plan was signed by both Mrs.
White and Jan, thereby establishing mutually agreed-on goals.

VNA

Name: Rose White   ID# _____

Date	Problem	Goal	Intervention	Date resolved
6/29	depressive symptoms interfere with self-care ability. AEB repeat hospital-izations	↓ depressive symptoms ↑ medical stability ↓ hospital visits	– Psychosocial Assessment 6/29 – Consult with psychiatrist re: Psy-chotropic meds 7/6 – develop self nurturing plan 6/29 – ↑ social support options – maximize natural coping mecha-nism 6/29 – Peer counselors referral? – Bereavement counseling re: multi-ple losses – Psycho Ed. regarding depressive symptoms	
6/29	medication non-compliance ↑ CHF symptoms	↑ Med compliance	– explore barriers to med compli-ance, i.e., passive suicidal behav-ior 6/29 – joint visit with nurses? – large calendar to check meds 6/29	
6/29	↓ weight (15 lb) in past month	return to at least baseline weight ↑ by 15 lbs	– assess barriers to adequate nutri-tion i.e. ↓ vision a factor? 6/29 – develop immediate plan to ↑ nu-trition support nursing suggestion of Ensure ? MOW every day ? enjoyable foods available 6/29 – Meals at Senior Center 6/29	
6/29	Level I suicide risk	↓ suicide risk	– Safety Plan - 6/29 – Emergency Services Alert 6/29 – Visit 2 × weekly × 2 weeks and re-evaluate	

MSW Signature: Date:

Please date and initial additions to the plan
Original—MSS Chart   Yellow—VN Chart

FIGURE 6.4   Case 1 MSS treatment plan (social work).

From: Visiting Nurse & Health Services. A program of Franklin Medical Center, Greenfield, MA. A member of Baystate Health Systems.

VNA

Name: Rose White   ID# _____

Date	Problem	Goal	Intervention	Date resolved
	Med Non-compliance	Med Compliance	– Education re: meds – Weekly prep of meds in pill box – ↓ frequency of daily doses TID → BID	
	↓ weight	↑ weight by 15 lbs	– evaluate for access to food – Nutrition education – MOW referral – Use of Ensure as supplement to food	
	depression	↓ depression	– Social Work Referral – evaluate for suicide risk – evaluate for med side effects – evaluate sleep patterns – physical assessment	

MSW Signature: _____   Date:

Please date and initial additions to the plan
Original—MSS Chart   Yellow—VN Chart

FIGURE 6.5   Case 1 nursing treatment plan.

From: Visiting Nurse & Health Services. A program of Franklin Medical Center, Greenfield, MA. A member of Baystate Health Systems.

Jan then addressed treatment issues as highlighted in the treatment plan (see Figures 6.4-Case 1, *Social Work Plan* and 6.5-Case 1, *Nursing Plan*). The dovetailing of the nursing and social work plans is quite apparent. Table 6.3 shows the contrasting, yet totally complementary, approaches in three major problem areas in Case 1, medication noncompliance, weight loss, and depression.

Emergency telephone numbers (visiting nurse association and emergency services) were reviewed and written in large numbers near the telephone. This crisis visit by Jan, which lasted 1 1/2 hours, assessed and addressed the passive suicidal behavior of this sad woman. The safety

TABLE 6.3   Social Worker–Nurse Approaches to Major Problems in Case 1

Social work activities	Nurse activities
Medication noncompliance	*Medication noncompliance*
1. Explore barriers to compliance (i. e., passive suicidal behavior)	1. Education re: medications
2. Joint visit with nurse	2. Weekly preparation of medications in a medication box
3. Large calendar to check meds	3. Decrease frequency of daily doses (3 to 2 times per day)
Weight loss	*Weight loss*
1. Assess barriers to adequate nutrition (e.g., loss of vision; decreased appetite secondary to depression)	1. Evaluate for access to food
2. Develop plan to increase nutrition support (take nursing suggestions re: nutrition supplements (Ensure & Meals on Wheels)	2. Nutrition education
3. Meals at Senior Center as a future goal	3. Meals on Wheels referral
	4. Use of Ensure as supplement to food
Depression	*Depression*
1. Psychosocial assessment	1. Social work referral
2. Consult with psychiatrist re: psychotropic medications	2. Evaluate for suicide risk
3. Develop self-nurturing-safety plan	3. Evaluate for medication side effects
4. Increase social support options	4. Evaluate sleep patterns
5. Maximize natural coping mechanism	5. Physical assessment
6. Peer counselor referral	
7. Bereavement counseling re: multiple losses	
8. Psychoeducation re: depressive symptoms	

plan integrates her significant strengths, her love of music, her ability to engage with others and integrate new information, and her devotion to her dog of 7 years. Jan will continue to work with Mrs. White to achieve medical and emotional stability. It is clear that the nurse–social worker team has meshed their assessments and action plans so that the unique and combined strengths of both professions are in full concert on behalf of Mrs. White.

Abuse/neglect screening for adults: ☐ None of the following observed/as-
                                                          sessed on this date

☐   1.   History/Evidence of domestic violence.
☐   2.   Suspicious physical injuries.
         (Bruises, lacerations or abrasions, head injuries and fractures: unexplained or
         disparate explanations; delays between injury/illness and seeking medical at-
         tention, frequent E.R. visits, etc.)
☑   3.   Clinical signs of neglect by others or self.
         (Dehydration, malnourishment, depression, withdrawal, anxiety, poor hy-
         giene, inadequate dress, etc.)
☑   4.   Caregiver issues.
         (Including substance abuse, mental illness, housing or finances shared with or
         dependent on patient. Overprotective of patient; does not leave patient alone
         with health worker.)
☑   5.   Patient/Caregiver stressors.
         (Bereavement, financial stress, or exacerbation of illness, etc.)

If any of the above are indicated, refer to MSS for evaluation.

FIGURE 6.6   Case 2 abuse screening.

From: Visiting Nurse & Health Services. A program of Franklin Medical Center,
Greenfield, MA. A member of Baystate Health Systems.

CASE 2: MR. JOHNSON

The second case example is a mandatory social work referral based on the
nursing Abuse and Neglect Screening protocol (see Figure 6.6-Case 2,
Abuse/Neglect Screening for Adults). The family constellation of a frail
parent and adult child can be problematic if the adult child is emotionally
unstable and financially dependent on the parent. Unfortunately, this is not
a rare situation. The potential risk for all involved, including the home
health care staff, is a reality in this particular case. The social worker, Jean,
is referred to assess safety concerns and to address identified problems that
interfere with the medical stability of the client (see Figure 6.7-Case 2,
Medical Social Services Referral).

Mr. Johnson was referred (as "high priority") for "COPD, CHF, oxygen
dependency, concerns re: nutrition, caregiver son shouting at home health
aide and client increase in emergency department visits." Requests for
services were in the areas of psychosocial assessment, life style change
due to disease, marital-family relationships, safety-environmental issues,
caregiver stress, frequent hospital visits or contacts, and abuse-neglect or

Patient: Joseph Johnson   DOB: _____ ID#: _____

Primary Care Physician _____ Other M.D. _____ SOP: _____

Disciplines Involved: ☑ VN ☑ HHA ☐ PT ☐ OT ☐ ST   Contact in home: Pt or: __

REASON FOR REFERRAL (check all that apply):   ☑ High Priority

☑ Psychosocial assessment   ☐ Health Care Proxy   ☐ Arrange for alternate living situation

☐ Community resource planning   ☑ Caregiver stress   ☑ Frequent hospital visits or contacts

☑ Life style change due to disease   ☐ Depression   ☐ QD or BID VN visits

☐ Medication/Tx non-compliance   ☐ Grief   ☑ Abuse/neglect or domestic violence indicators

☑ Marital/family relationships   ☐ Finances

☑ Safety/environmental issues   ☐ Substance abuse

Other: COPD, CHF, oxygen dependent, concerns re: nutrition. Caregiver son shouts at HHA and client. Recent increase in Emergency Department visits

Referred by: _____   Date: _____ Projected duration of VN Service: _____

MSS Form 1 4/96   Medication Profile and Nursing Narratives are attached.

FIGURE 6.7   Case 2 medical social services referral.

From: Visiting Nurse & Health Services. A program of Franklin Medical Center, Greenfield, MA. A member of Baystate Health Systems.

domestic violence indicators. An elder protective service report may be made depending on the results of the social work assessment.

Case 2 will be divided into its major components of nurse–social worker collaboration, as for Case 1. These are abuse and neglect; safety of the nurses, social workers, and home health aides going into this home; nutrition; anxiety about medical condition; and depression (see Figures 6.8-Case 2, *Social Work Plan* and 6.9-Case 2, *Nursing Plan*).

Home health care social work within volatile systems, such as with this client, demands an advanced level of social work skills, a high level of teamwork, and active supervision. The client in this case is very defended and fearful of interventions that may escalate his caregiver's hostility. His ultimate fear is nursing home placement in the event that his son becomes unwilling or unable to care for him in his home. Generational

VNA

Name: Joseph Johnson   ID# _____

Date	Problem	Goal	Intervention	Date resolved
2/8	Indicators of domestic conflict & concerns regarding worker (HHA) & client safety	↓ conflict in home → safe environment for client and worker	– Assessment of client & caregiver system especially re: safety, issues – develop safety plan for client & workers – Multi-provider case conference – Call Protective Service if indicated – Lifeline referral ASAP – Assess caregivers stress – ↑ Home Health services? – phone beside client chair ASAP	
2/8	Concerns re: nutrition ↑ weight may ↑ general strength & ↑ pleasure	↑ weight by 10–15 lbs	– explore barriers to ↑ nutrition i.e. depression. – HHA to prepare PM meal? – ? conflict during meal time	
2/8	Client anxiety re: (lack of Advance Directive & incomplete will) = ↑ COPD symptoms	↓ anxiety	– Ed re advance directives – meeting with client and identified Health Care agent – completion of A.D. – Speak with client's Attorney re: will & need to complete at home	
2/8	depressed mood may interfere with ability to care for self	Assess & address depressed mood if indicated	– Psycho-Social Assessment – Engage client to ↓ defenses with writer – Short term therapy if indicated especially re: losses	

MSW Signature: Date:

Please date and initial additions to the plan
Original—MSS Chart   Yellow—VN Chart

FIGURE 6.8   Case 2 MSS treatment plan (social work).

From: Visiting Nurse & Health Services. A program of Franklin Medical Center, Greenfield, MA. A member of Baystate Health Systems.

VNA

Name: Joseph Johnson   ID# _____

Date	Problem	Goal	Intervention	Date resolved
12/29	Inadequate nutrition—10–15 lbs under base-line weight	↑ wt. by 10–15 lbs	– consult with M.D. – evaluate for access to food – MOW referral – referral for services from Elder Services – weight 2 × weekly – nutrition education	
2/8	↑ concerns re: possible verbal abuse & neglect by caregiver son.	Assess and respond to A&N concerns	– Social Work Referral—high priority 2/8	
2/8	Concerns regarding safety of HHAs in home	Safe work environment for HHAs	– Consult with HHA Supervisor & other HHAs in case 2/8 – Consult with Social Work Supervisor & Nurse Manager 2/8	

MSW Signature: Date:

Please date and initial additions to the plan
Original—MSS Chart   Yellow—VN Chart

FIGURE 6.9   Case 2 nursing treatment plan.

From: Visiting Nurse & Health Services. A program of Franklin Medical Center, Greenfield, MA. A member of Baystate Health Systems.

mores regarding family privacy challenge the social worker in her attempt to engage the client and the caregiver. In some cases, limit-setting with the caregiver may require the nurse and social worker to assume a good cop–bad cop dynamic with the social worker in the latter role. The good role protects the nurse's opportunity to continue her nursing functions. Safety plans in this case are developed by both team members but monitored by the social worker (Table 6.4).

Mr. Johnson is cognitively high functioning and insists on continued care at home by his son. The client's agenda is accepted by the social worker and directs her work in this case. She attempts to align with the

TABLE 6.4   Approaches to Major Problems in Case 2

Social work activities	Nurse activities
Abuse and neglect/worker safety	*Abuse and neglect/work safety*
1. Assessment of client and caregiver system (especially re: safety issues)	1. Social work referral—high priority
2. Develop safety plan for client and workers	2. Consult with home health aide and social work supervisors; nurse manager re: safety of home health aides in home
3. Multi-provider case conference	
4. Call protective service if indicated	
5. Lifeline referral as soon as possible	
6. Assess caregiver's stress and strengths	
7. Increase home health services	
8. Phone beside client chair as soon as possible	
Nutrition	*Nutrition*
1. Explore barriers to better nutrition (i. e., depression)	1. Consult with physician
2. Home health aide to prepare evening meal	2. Evaluate for access to food
3. Question conflict during meal time	3. Meals on Wheels referral
	4. Referral for services from Elder Services
	5. Check weight 2 times weekly
	6. Nutrition education
Anxiety about medical condition	*Anxiety about medical condition*
1. Assess sources of anxiety	1. Education re: medical condition management
2. Education re: advance directives and incomplete will	
3. Meeting with client and identified health care agent	
4. Completing of advance directive	
5. Speak with client's attorney re: will and need to complete at home	
Depression	*Depression*
1. Psychosocial assessment	1. Social work referral
2. Engage client to lower defenses	2. Assess for medication side effects
3. Short-term therapy, if indicated, especially re: losses	

son to both limit-set and to support his caregiver role. The treatment plans are developed to define both social work and nurse interventions. Clear delineation of both roles is essential, especially in cases involving interpersonal conflict between client and family or others.

The dramatic shift of health care provision from acute care settings to the community and home environments has triggered tremendous national growth in home health care services delivery. This is usually accomplished by nurses and social workers in teams. The model is health and behavioral health care for the entire life span that is relevant, available, and accessible. In some home health organizations nurses and social workers experience tension secondary to unclear role definition. The development of social work protocols and practice guidelines that reflect the clinical work unique to social work can assist in the creation of dynamic nurse–social work teams. Communication will also be enhanced. The collision of major medical and psychosocial stressors is the norm in home health care work. Experienced collaborative nurse–social work teams offer a powerful, holistic response to these complex cases in the community.

REFERENCES

Kulys, R., & Davis, M. A. Sr. (1987). Nurses and social workers: Rivals in the provision of services? *Health and Social Work, 12*, 101–111.

National Association of Social Workers. (1992). *Standards of Social Work Case Management*. Annapolis Junction, MD: NASW Press.

Nursing and Social Work Case Documentation. (1996). Greenfield, MA: Franklin Medical Center, Visiting Nurse Association and Health Services.

CHAPTER 7

A Flexible, Community-Based Approach to Assessment, Diagnosis, and Outcomes Measurement

The proposed Biopsychosocial Individual and Systems Intervention Model (BISIM) calls for new assessment and diagnostic indicators and parameters. Assessment in health and behavioral health determines initial goals and the evaluation, at some subsequent point, of their success or failure of accomplishment (Callahan, 1996). Assessment should be ongoing. Assessment, therefore, focuses the beginning, flexibly informs the ongoing intervention process, and provides outcome benchmarks for accountability in all health and behavioral health interventions. As such, assessment must contain relevant, reliable, and valid initial indicators. These indicators must also be couched in terms that are easily understood by all members of the intervention team.

Broadly conceived health and risk-assessment measurement tools are needed. These must be community based determined and calibrated by more than one professional group, and informed by much more than the traditional illness-pathology models in a clinical model of intervention. Protocols linking problem assessments, focused interventions, flexible changes in approach during a person's life span (the time-frame posited for the BISIM), and delineation of expected and desired outcomes are essential. Finally, the constraining yoke of the strictly clinical model (both medical and psychiatric) of diagnosis and intervention must be thrown off in favor of a community-based model, which does not see the world through the eyes of either an institution (such as hospital or social welfare bureaucracy, which entrapped both nursing and social work for 50 years) or a single professional group (such as physicians or psychologists).

The new community care model, which is both enabled and constrained by managed care systems, is extraordinarily complex. Old health institutional systemic supports, with their comforting and annoying structures, rigidities, and hierarchical control from the top of the system, are giving way to a more flexible multidisciplinary team of professional equals approach in the community. This is why a flexible, community-based diagnostic and assessment taxonomy is essential. The old ones do not inform current or future community health and behavioral health practice. They must, therefore, be modified, qualified, expanded, or abandoned altogether. This can only be accomplished by the team in the community, in this case, collaborating nurses and social workers.

LIMITATIONS OF OLD PATHOLOGY-BASED ASSESSMENT AND DIAGNOSTIC MODELS

The establishment of jointly agreed-on assessment indicators and instruments to capture these indicators reliably and with validity is at once the most important and difficult for the nurse–social worker collaborative team. Mutual language reflective of commonly understood concepts, roles, and techniques is the cornerstone of team communication. As was discussed in chapter 5, communication problems are powerful predictors of difficulties in nurse–social worker collaboration.

To compound basic communication problems, commonly employed diagnostic and assessment categories are frequently both too narrow and too vague to be useful guides for service interventions. This is particularly true for social work, which has, due to lack of diagnostic and intervention protocols (which are ubiquitous in the nursing field), become dependent on diagnostic taxonomies for practice designed by other professions (most notably psychiatry and psychology) that do not relate to actual social work practice or systematically exclude common social work interventions as appropriate for reimbursement by managed care companies. Such is the case with the *Diagnostic and Statistical Manual of Mental Disorders* (DSM-IV), in particular, the V Section.

This chapter will discuss three intertwined issues in relation to assessment and diagnosis as they pertain to nurse–social worker collaboration in the community: (a) the narrowness of current assessment and diagnostic tools and categories, especially such taxonomies as *DSM-IV* and medical diagnoses, for broadly based work in the community; (b) fallacies, unreliabilities, and invalidities of existing psychiatric assessment and diagnostic categories; (c) ethics, cultural and gender sensitivities, and diagnosis.

NARROWNESS OF CURRENT ASSESSMENT AND DIAGNOSTIC TOOLS AND CATEGORIES

The category of "Other Conditions That May Be a Focus of Clinical Attention" (the "V Section") in the American Psychiatric Association's *Diagnostic Criteria from DSM-IV* (1994) is excluded from reimbursement by managed care companies (Jackson, 1995). These 31 excluded conditions are listed in Table 7.1.

Except for the eight medication-induced categories, the other 23 areas are precisely where social work performs the bulk of its interventions, both within institutions and in the community. Further, these areas of functioning are those of primary concern to community health and behavioral health efforts during the entire life span. These are the very areas that will be of crucial concern in the proposed BISIM of nurse–social worker collaborative services delivery in the community.

Strictly medical diagnoses are crucial for physical illness assessment and provide one basis for nursing protocols. In the area of psychosocial behavioral health, however, such diagnostic frameworks as *DSM-IV* are unreliable, frequently invalid, and far too narrowly restricted to purely psychological (and, lingeringly, psychoanalytic) pathological factors. What is crucial to assessment in the community, but totally missing in *DSM-IV* (and excluded from insurance reimbursement when present) are those psychosocial problems in living that are focused on psychosocial functional levels in the family, work group, school, and community. Interventions deriving from these problems in living assessment areas must be grounded in client strengths and competencies.

FALLACIES, UNRELIABILITIES, AND INVALIDITIES OF EXISTING PSYCHIATRIC ASSESSMENT AND DIAGNOSTIC CATEGORIES

Fallacies, unreliabilities, and invalidities of existing psychiatric assessment and diagnostic categories pertain only to the behavioral health area because this is the area for which these categories were designed and promulgated. Numerous studies have pointed to unreliability and lack of validity in these assessment and diagnostic categories. If they are unreliable, they are, by definition, invalid. If they are either or both, they are false. If they are false, then they are, at best, unhelpful and, at worst, harmful to at-risk and stressed clients and patients who need help (Kirk & Kutchins, 1992).

TABLE 7.1   Conditions That May Be a Focus of Clinical Attention

Eight medication-induced movement disorders

- neuroleptic-induced parkinsonism
- malignant syndrome
- acute dystonia
- acute akathisia
- tardive dyskinesia
- postural tremor
- medication-induced movement
- disorder not otherwise specified
- adverse effects of medication not otherwise specified

Relational problems

V61.9	Relational problems related to a mental disorder or general medical condition
V61.20	Parent-child relational problem
V61.1	Partner relational problem
V61.8	Sibling relational problem
V62.81	Relational problem not otherwise specified

Problems related to abuse and neglect

V61.21	Physical abuse of child
V61.21	Sexual abuse of child
V61.21	Neglect of child
V61.1	Physical abuse of adult
V61.1	Sexual abuse of adult

Additional conditions that may be a focus of clinical attention

V15.81	Noncompliance with treatment
V65.2	Malingering
V71.01	Adult antisocial behavior
V71.02	Child or adolescent antisocial behavior
V62.89	Borderline intellectual functioning
780.9	Age-related cognitive decline
V62.82	Bereavement
V62.3	Academic problem
V62.2	Occupational problem
313.82	Identity problem
V62.89	Religious or spiritual problem
V62.4	Acculturation problem
V62.89	Phase of life problem (pp. 287–301).

From: American Psychiatric Association. (1994). *Diagnostic and Statistical Manual of Mental Disorders* (4th ed.). Washington, DC: American Psychiatric Press.

ETHICS, CULTURAL AND GENDER SENSITIVITIES, AND DIAGNOSES: MANAGED CARE OFF-BASE

Managed care companies are under almost constant fire not only for their rigid reliance on narrow and frequently unhelpful *DSM-IV* psychiatric diagnoses, but for playing fast and loose with both medical and psychiatric data in their computer systems. A recent example is a managed care company leaking preexisting conditions such as HIV/AIDS status to employers, thus prompting an employee to be fired. Employee assistance programs in corporate settings and the social work profession as a whole have labored to maintain the ethical tenet of confidentiality, only to have managed care companies utilize and disseminate predominately unreliable and invalid categories.

Another example is the all too frequently applied *DSM-IV* label, 301.83 "Borderline Personality Disorder," described as "a pervasive pattern of instability of interpersonal relationships, self-image, and affects, and marked impulsivity beginning by early adulthood and present in a variety of contexts . . . " (American Psychiatric Association, 1994, p. 280). This almost incomprehensibly broad description is frequently shared with persons in the community whose appropriateness to receive such information is questionable.

Diagnostic categories as inflexible and theory-bound as the *DSM-IV* are bound to run into cultural relevance problems. Kirmayer (1994) argued persuasively that it is not only the boundaries and definitions of disorder that differ across cultures, but that "the concept of 'mental disorder' itself is a creation of Western cultural history for which no exact parallel can be found in many other traditions" (p. 2). He made the point that three of the medical traditions of the world (Islamic, Ayurvedic, and Chinese) "treat the person as a psychophysical unity and so make no fundamental distinction between mental and physical illness" (p. 5). In other words, these world-view traditions have no language (and, presumably, no corresponding mental concepts) to represent the mind-body split so popular in Western thought.

Kirmayer's main point was summarized as follows: " . . . many problems in other cultures (and perhaps in our own) that current nosology attempts to construct as discreet disorders are not deviant or disorders at all. They are culturally constituted and sanctioned *idioms of distress*—vocabularies and styles for explaining and expressing a wide range of personal and social problems. These idioms of distress cannot simply be added to our lists of discrete entities. Instead, they must be understood as rhetorical devices for making sense of human predicaments" (p. 7).

Not only is the diagnostic issue potentially unethical and fraught with the possibility of cultural misinterpretations, but it is sexist. Not surprisingly, women make up the vast majority of those diagnosed with ''borderline personality disorder.'' In a polemic article in the press, Madeline Drexler took on *DSM-IV* for its rampant and invidious sexist view of the ''mentally ill, psychologically dysfunctional, or, in the world's eyes, crazy'' (Drexler, 1995, p. 3). Further, ''with its decimal-point coding, starched prose, and 3-pound heft, the *DSM* has an unmistakable air of authority. It should, since mental-health professionals and physicians rely on it for their diagnoses, insurers use it for reimbursement, and courts cite it in legal decisions. But far from being empirically grounded, the *DSM* is permeated with shoddy science and value judgments . . . '' (p. 4).

There are predominantly (or exclusively) women's illnesses, such as Self-Defeating Personality Disorder (originally Masochistic Personality Disorder) and Premenstrual Dysphoric Disorder. Self-Defeating Personality Disorder was dropped from the current *DSM-IV*, but Premenstrual Dysphoric Disorder was not. The point is that ''the *DSM* is more likely to pathologize women's socially shaped behavior than men's'' (Drexler, 1995, p. 4).

AN ASSESSMENT AND DIAGNOSTIC FRAMEWORK FOR THE NURSE–SOCIAL WORKER COLLABORATIVE TEAM

The preferred assessment and diagnostic framework is the client strengths model, modified by other factors. The basic assumption for any diagnostic and assessment model is that it proceed from a strengths and coping basis rather than a sickness-weakness and pathology set of baseline measures.

Cowger pointed out that ''social work has been long on philosophy and theory that flaunts a client strength perspective, but short on practice directives, guidelines, and know-how for incorporating strengths into practice'' (1992, p. 139). The so-called strengths school has a long history in social work. Maluccio, one of its major initiators and proponents, has argued persuasively for a shift in social work from ''problems or pathology to strengths, resources, and potentialities in human beings and their environments'' (1981, p. 401). The term *assessment* is preferred to *diagnosis* because it is more in line with client strengths. The term diagnosis presupposes pathology in both the physical and behavioral health areas. The assessment framework most appropriate for nurse–social work team collaboration is one that initially assesses, and works with throughout the life span, the strengths of individuals, groups, communities, and organizations.

The strengths model enhances nurse–social worker communication because it is a common one both in initial training and subsequent practice for both professions. This is not the case for most of the other psychosocial models, especially ones that are based on psychodynamic theory. Cowger's assessment process consists of two components: defining the problem situation and framework for assessment (1992, pp. 141–146).

DEFINING THE PROBLEM SITUATION (OR GETTING AT WHY THE CLIENT SEEKS ASSISTANCE)

1. Brief summary of the identified problem situation (should be in simple language, straightforward, and mutually agreed on by worker and client. It can be no more than a brief paragraph);
2. Who (persons, groups, or organizations) is involved including the client(s) seeking assistance?
3. How or in what way are participants involved? What happens between the participants before, during, and immediately following activity related to the problem situation?
4. What meaning does the client ascribe to the problem situation?
5. What does the client want in relation to the problem situation?
6. What does the client want or expect by seeking assistance?
7. What would the client's life be like if the problem was resolved?

FRAMEWORK FOR ASSESSMENT

This assessment component involves analyzing, evaluating, and giving meaning to these factors that influence the problem situation. It also involves the design of an action intervention plan. Cowger's framework has four axes for assessment (Figure 7.1).

Cowger also has a lengthy list for assessment of client strengths (pp. 144–147). The Cowger model may provide a useful framework for thinking about the appropriateness and inclusiveness of some of the assessment tools discussed below.

Several authors have discussed assessment (Carlton, 1984; Feldman & Fitzpatrick, 1992; Maluccio, 1981; Surber, 1994; Vourlekis & Greene, 1992). None posited a framework specific enough to be immediately useful for nurse–social worker team practice.

Other assessment tools have been recently discussed (Van Hook, Berkman, & Dunkle, 1996). The three assessment tools for general health care settings, Primary Care Evaluation of Mental Health Disorders (PRIME-MD), Older Americans Resources and Services Questionnaire (OARS),

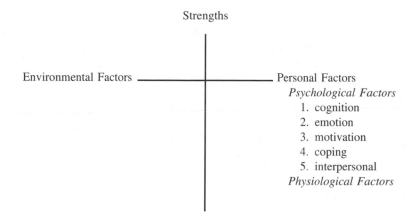

FIGURE 7.1   Assessment axes.

and Health-Related Quality-of-Life Measure (HRQL), suggested by the authors are for different populations. All are useful assessment tools because, when taken together, their applicability is wide by virtue of health and behavioral health category and age grouping.

PRIME-MD was designed to diagnose mental health problems in the primary care sector. OARS was designed to provide functional assessments essential for effective clinical management of elderly clients. The point is well taken that there is increasing evidence that clinicians are not good at predicting a patient's functional abilities (Elam et al., 1989). Of the three instruments, the HRQL appears to hold the most promise for nurse–social work interventions in the community setting.

The HRQL focuses attention on quality-of-life outcomes that are important to patients themselves, not only to those professionals doing the assessing. The patient or client, therefore, is placed squarely at the center of the whole process. "It is virtually impossible with existing knowledge to determine what effects most social work services, such as family conferences, have on patient-level outcomes or whether the effect is preferable to the outcomes that may have resulted from other services being given (such as peer groups) or from no services being given. It has thus become imperative for social work professionals to begin conducting outcome research using measures that reflect functional quality-of-life outcomes" (Van Hook et al., 1996, p. 232).

In the past health and behavioral health assessment and outcome measures have been narrowly defined, based on traditional clinical indices, as has been pointed out. The HRQL, developed as part of the Medical Outcomes Study at the New England Medical Center in Boston with assistance from the Rand Corporation in Santa Monica, California, is potentially useful because it is based on a "new paradigm that health care should be based and evaluated not just on its impact on morbidity and mortality, but also on how patients view its effect on their quality of life" (Van Hook et al., 1996, p. 233). It is just these functional quality-of-life outcomes that both social workers and nurses (and all others on the team) must measure as indicators of successful interventions in a wide variety of situations and over the entire life span.

REFERENCES

American Psychiatric Association. (1994). *Diagnostic criteria from DSM-IV*. Washington, DC: Author.

Callahan, J. (1996). Documentation of client dangerousness in a managed care environment. *Health and Social Work, 21*, 202–207.

Carlton, T. O. (1984). *Clinical social work in health settings. A guide to professional practice with exemplars*. New York: Springer.

Cowger, C. D. (1992). Assessment of client strengths. In D. Saleebey (Ed.), *The strengths perspective in social work practice* (pp. 139–147). White Plains, NY: Longman.

Drexler, M. (1995). Deciding who's normal. *Boston Globe Magazine*, July 9, 6.

Elam, J., Beaver, T., El Derwi, D., Applegate, W., Graney, M., & Miller, S. (1989). Comparison of sources of functional report with observed functional ability of frail older persons. *Gerontologist, 29*(Suppl.), 308A.

Feldman, J. L., & Fitzpatrick, R. J. (Eds.). (1992). *Managed mental health care. Administrative and clinical issues*. Washington, DC: American Psychiatric Press.

Jackson, V. H. (Ed.). (1995). *Managed care resource guide—Agency settings*. Annapolis Junction, MD: NASW Press.

Kirk, S. A., & Kutchins, H. (1992). *The selling of DSM. The rhetoric of science in psychiatry*. New York: Aldine De Gruyter.

Kirmayer, L. J. (1994). Is the concept of mental disorder culturally relative? Yes. In S. A. Kirk & S. D. Enbinder (Eds.), *Controversial issues in mental health* (pp. 1–11). Boston: Allyn and Bacon.

Maluccio, A. N. (Ed.). (1981). *Promoting competence in clients. A new/old approach to social work practice*. New York: Free Press.

Saleebey, D. (1992). *The strengths perspective in social work practice*. White Plains, NY: Longman.

Surber, R. W. (1994). *Clinical case management. A guide to comprehensive treatment of serious mental illness*. Thousand Oaks, CA: Sage.

Van Hook, M. P., Berkman, B., & Dunkle, R. (1996). Assessment tools for general health care settings: PRIME-MD, OARS, and SF-36. *Health and Social Work, 21*, 230–234.

Vourlekis, B. S., & Greene, R. R. (Eds.). (1992). *Social work case management*. New York: Aldine De Gruyter.

CHAPTER 8

The Hospital View

Valerie A. Hamel

The creation of an open market in health care has caused an unprecedented transformation in the way hospitals operate. In the 1980s, hospitals were singled out in an attempt to control skyrocketing health care costs. As a result, hospitals have changed the way they deliver health care. The impact that these hospital changes have had on nursing and social work will be the major focus of this chapter. Exploring what new opportunities lie ahead, in and out of the hospital, for the two professions will also be discussed. Although it is not the intent of this chapter to detail the specifics of hospital bureaucracy, it is necessary to review them. This will allow us to proceed to the more relevant task of determining how these will affect the future of nursing and social work.

THE HOSPITAL IS NO LONGER THE QUARTERBACK

Managed care has altered many typical hospital practices. Chamberlain, Chen, Osuna, and Yamamoto (1995) cleverly captured the hospital structure before managed care came onto the playing field. They noted that for decades payment for health care was based on fee for services. This system provided health care providers little incentive to monitor for wasteful and unnecessary services and greatly contributed to the soaring costs of health care. Hospitals and physicians benefitted from this setup, as revenues and profits continued to increase. Physicians were the driving force of hospitals, in that they selected the institution for patients. Whether the services were necessary or appropriate wasn't of much concern to the hospital.

This behavior continued unchecked for some time before Medicare instituted a prospective payment system to control exacerbating costs.

111

This system was based on a diagnosis-related group (DRG) design. DRGs were developed at Yale University in 1983 and became a basis for payment for Medicare patients in the 1980s. The admission diagnosis placed the patient in a particular DRG. Payments were made according to the set fee based on the DRG assigned. Chamberlain et al. (1995, p. 232) stated "For the first time, hospitals had a reason to regulate their own efficiency." This was the beginning of managed care's influence over hospitals.

It was about this same time that the Joint Commission on Accreditation of Hospitals, known now as the Joint Commission on Accreditation of Healthcare Organizations, began to require that the appropriateness of hospital services be examined. Hospitals would now have to be accountable for their actions if they wanted to maintain their accreditation.

A NEW PLAYING FIELD

A large portion of the U.S. population now receives health care through managed care organizations. Bostrom reported (1995) that there are now more than 1,000 managed care firms providing health insurance to employees in the United States. If hospitals want to provide services to patients covered by particular managed care organizations, they need to contract with them and play by their rules. Because of the numerous managed care firms, there has been a scramble among many hospitals to contract with any and all managed care organizations to maintain a competitive edge. It seems some hospitals are so desperate for ever-shrinking health care dollars, they (hospitals) are willingly to accept any offer managed care throws their way.

Many industry observers believe this behavior has produced a number of obstacles that hospitals are struggling to overcome. "The administrative burden placed on a hospital involved in numerous managed care agreements can be substantial," stated Lewis (1992, p. 15). In many instances around the country, hospitals are involved with contractual relationships with multiple managed care organizations.

With these multiple contract arrangements came more and more managed care organizations dictating what hospital services would be covered (Harrington & Estes, 1994). Health insurance often differs from company to company, both in coverage and the processing requirements. Variations in coverage are based on details of specific employer-managed insurance contracts. For example, it is fairly common for some managed care insurance to require preauthorization for a hospital admission or any diagnostic testing and denial of payment if the appropriate forms and authorization numbers are not used; still another might have very detailed agreements regarding length of stay (LOS), and so on. As a result, the variation in coverage and processing detail is usually several times greater than the number of contracts alone (Bostrom, 1995). Indeed, the age of managed care has forced hospitals to deal with very complex and costly issues associated with furnishing health care services.

Along with managed care, there has also been a dramatic shift in ownership of hospitals from the public sector to nonprofit and for-profit organizations. Nonprofit and for-profit hospitals are supposed to balance each other with regard to community support: Nonprofit hospitals continue to provide charity care to the poor and in return they are tax-exempt; and for-profit hospitals pay the usual taxes that other businesses pay, thus the community benefits from a tax-paying business.

Membership among these organizations has also changed in the past few years; for-profit organizations have gained substantial yardage over their nonprofit counterparts. White (1995) reported that in 1988 for-profit member plans had a total enrollment of 15.4 million people, whereas nonprofit plans had 17.2 million members. By 1993, total enrollment in for-profit plans had grown dramatically to 24.8 million people, whereas nonprofit plans were providing care to 20.4 million people.

According to Burda (1995), there are many critics of the for-profit organizations. The critics accuse for-profit investors, particularly Columbia/HCA Healthcare Corporation, the nation's largest investor-owned hospital chain, of being on a mission driven by making money for stockholders and not community need. Burda (1995) reported the response from a for-profit hospital representative was "stockholders make the world go around" (p. 28). The for-profit hospital owners have also been accused of limiting hospital services, closing down hospitals not making a profit, or both. Their representatives deny these allegations.

Hospital mergers are common within these organizations. Many hospital mergers (also known as horizontal integration) have resulted in the formation of huge multihospital systems. These systems in turn are becoming consolidated, with large companies controlling the largest share of the overall hospital market (Harrington & Estes, 1994).

Vertical integration is another way that large enterprises are buying their way into the health care market. Harrington and Estes (1994) defined vertical integration as the development of organizations with different levels and types of services. For instance, a company may own or contract with physicians, hospitals, pharmacies, nursing homes, surgicenters, and insurance companies. If any of these services are required, referrals are made within the organization. According to Greene (1995), of the nation's 6,467 hospitals in 1993, 44% were owned, leased, or managed by multihospital healthcare systems.

Greene (1995b) also reported that hospitals that are part of a multihospital system are more likely to receive the Joint Commission on Accreditation of Healthcare Organizations' highest recognition, accreditation with commendation. Accreditation and commendation recognize a hospital's exemplary performance in areas such as quality improvement, patients' rights, medication use, practitioner credentialing, safety, and organizational management. This may give hospitals with accreditation an important advantage in managed care contracting in the future. Thus, hospitals are provided with yet another incentive to allow investor-owned organizations to take over their institutions.

LEARNING TO BE A TEAM MEMBER IN AND OUT OF THE HOSPITAL

With the preceding discussion in mind, we are now ready to explore what has happened to the professions of nursing and social work within the hospital. First, we will tackle how managed care has affected nurses in the hospital setting. Next, we will examine some steps taken by the nursing discipline in response to hospitals controlled by managed care. We will then focus our attention on the profession of social work and examine how managed care is directing its future.

NURSES IN HOSPITALS IN THE 1990S

As mentioned earlier, hospitals are now run like many other businesses. The name of the game is providing high quality care, while at the same time being as cost effective as possible. For many hospitals, this has meant downsizing and eliminating departments and staff considered nonessential.

Most would agree that one of the departments hardest hit by these actions is the nursing department, particularly registered nurses (RNs). According to Huston (1996), the hospital staff composition of RNs has rapidly decreased from 90% just a few years ago to 69% in 1994. The reason most commonly cited for this decline is the increased utilization of unlicensed assistive personnel (UAP). Fagin and Gordon (1996) reported that hospitals hire high-priced consultants or administrators whose principal goal is determining how to cut cost by laying off RNs and replacing them with UAP.

The primary argument given by the hospitals for using UAP in acute-care settings is efficiency; UAP can free professional nurses from tasks and assignments that can be completed by less well-trained personnel at a lower cost, specifically, nonnursing functions. There are data that support this argument, noting that many nonclinical and patient-related activities done by nurses can be accomplished by secretaries, housekeepers, transporters, or other ancillary personnel (Huston, 1996).

Critics claim that several studies have concluded nurses' dissatisfaction increases as the number of nonnursing functions that they are required to do increases. Yet, nurses continue to debate the use of UAP to do such duties. The question put to nurses by advocates of UAP is: Why do nurses feel so threatened by their use?

Huston (1996) responded by citing some of nursing's concerns associated with UAP: (a) the training of the UAP is inadequate, especially considering the acuity of patients seen in the hospital today, (b) the added responsibility that dwindling numbers of RNs must assume in supervising UAP, (c) concern that the RN might not be properly trained to supervise UAP, (d) the fact that consumers (patients) are many times completely unaware that UAP are providing their care, and (e) the widely accepted premise that UAP utilization models have been proven cost efficient as well as safe.

Keepnews, director of policy for the American Nurses Association (ANA), asserted "Unlike the nursing home sector, where nursing assistants' responsibilities are generally agreed upon, one of the big problems in hospitals is the rapid expansion of unlicensed persons' responsibilities, often including functions that they cannot perform safely and reliably" (1996a, p. 5). Similar sentiments have been expressed by many observers.

Many of these concerns were recently reported to the Institute of Medicine's (IOM) Commission on the Adequacy of Nurse Staffing by the ANA. The IOM expressed its amazement regarding the hospital's lack of data in the implementation of such care. The IOM has called for research on hospital quality, on usable nursing workforce data, and on nurses' contribution to patient care outcomes (Keepnews, 1996b). To the disappointment of the ANA, no conclusion will be reached on this matter until the research has been completed and analyzed.

OFFENSIVE STRATEGIES

Whether one agrees with the present use of UAP, one needs to admit that changes in the hospital are probably going to continue. If the profession of nursing intends to remain a vital part of the health care team, it must prepare itself for the hospital of today and tomorrow. The nurse who is perspicacious about what is going on in the hospital setting can plan for the future. A major question for nursing staff is: How can I provide nursing care in the restructured environment? Nurses have to know the health care business and focus on their unique role in providing cost-effective, quality patient services. Cost-effectiveness and quality care are important in nursing care, and both are key to nursing's future in the hospital setting (Wieczorek, 1996).

Porter-O'Grady, an Atlanta-based consultant specializing in organizational transformation and health services reform, recommended that nurses get involved with the development of new health care models coming from the managed care market. According to Porter-O'Grady (1994), successful designs are those that result in more efficient and effective patient care. They start with certain principles and strategies. Here are a few questions that should help determine if a design will support cost-effective, quality care (Porter-O'Grady, 1994, p. 35):

• Is the model aimed at enhancing patient care, not just cutting cost?
• Does the new structure being created by the model reflect consultation with nurses and other professional care givers before planning and implementation?
• Does the consulting group include nurse-consultants? Is the nurse's role clearly defined in the context of coordinating, integrating, supporting, and assisting in the delivery of care, not simply by tasks or functions?
• Will the care team under the new structure be a partnership, with each member having a fair say in delineating responsibilities? Or, are responsibilities to be imposed by administrators, consultants, or advisors?
• Does the ratio of caregivers to patients systematically take into account care needs? Has it been determined in advance of the new design and evaluated to make sure it allows safe and effective patient care with reasonable workloads?

The demand for more outpatient and community-based care has resulted in an increase in opportunities for all nurses, including those known as advanced practice nurses (APN). Nurses in advanced practice (nurse practitioners, nurse-midwives, clinical nurse specialists, and certified registered nurse anesthetists), fit nicely within the managed care model. Studies cited in Safriet's (1992) extensively documented treatise, which supports changes in regulations to permit APNs to practice to the full extent of their preparation, underscored the cost-effectiveness of using APNs in providing care to many segments of the population. The fact that nurses can provide primary care of high quality, and some would argue a superior quality, for a lower cost than physicians, has managed care organizations seeking their services.

Reimbursement for nursing services has begun to allow for more independent practice and should improve the quality of care by improving access. Direct payment to APNs recognizes them as independent health care practitioners. This puts APNs on an equal footing with other practitioners who are paid directly for their services. Direct payment also provides recognition for APNs as unique providers in the health care system (Harrington & Estes, 1994).

In the past, nursing practice has focused on processes, failing to acknowledge the outcome-driven nature of health care. Nurses have been socialized into a system in which they lack power to develop health care delivery patterns and are sheltered from the impact of health care decisions because of the places they hold in the delivery system. Passive acceptance of managed care systems will only cause further problems associated with this role (Harrigan, 1995). With new health care design systems quickly developing within managed care hospitals, nurses need to make sure they are not left sitting on the sidelines again.

SOCIAL WORKERS IN HOSPITALS IN THE 1990S

Just as nurses are struggling under the current hospital climate of downsizing, introduction of UAP, and closing of units, social workers, too, feel the hot breath of managed care (or its results) on their necks. Rayburn and Rayburn wrote in 1996 that a shift in power has occurred to hospital accountants. As health care professionals, social workers join their colleagues in voicing their concern for clients whose needs may be subsumed in deference to the bottom line. What then does this shift of power, or those proposed by others from health care professionals to payers or for-profit health care conglomerates, mean to social workers whose careers have been in acute care?

In a study published in 1996, the authors painted a portrait of hospital social work in the 1990s similar to that of hospital nursing (Berger, et al., 1996). Decreased lengths of stay and decreasing occupancy rates and numbers of acute care beds were interpreted to mean that patients are moving through the hospital system at much faster rates, and competition for inpatient care has become more acute. As hospitals restructure, departments are being combined and management levels are being eliminated. Hospitals are developing new products: ambulatory services, establishing or linking up with community-based services, creating a continuum of care through affiliations with subacute and extended-care facilities, and home care agencies. Social workers are becoming involved in increasing numbers in community-based programs. Social workers in this study reported either increased clinical activity on inpatient units or no change. The net result of the question about staffing in hospital social work departments was no change; some departments are increasing, some decreasing, and some staying the same. Some concern was expressed by the study respondents over the hiring of nurses in social work departments, particularly for discharge planning, but the data did not bear this out (Berger, et al., 1996). However, a general sense of unrest colored by anecdotal reports, some of which did not bear out in the Berger et al. study, seems to characterize all of health care and the world of practice for social workers in particular.

OFFENSIVE STRATEGIES

The director of a social work department in a major teaching hospital put it this way: " . . . I face the challenge of continuing to be not only innovative in patient care services and program planning, but also flexible in our roles and relationships in order to meet a world where technology and economics evolve faster than we can describe" (Mayer, 1995, p. 71). Dimond and Markowitz (1995), reflecting on this rapidity of change and its impact on care delivery in acute care hospitals, observed that social workers need to market their social work expertise and the positive impact of social work practice on patient satisfaction if hospital social work departments are to survive. The departments must also "transform and mold service delivery . . . in harmony with the strategic plans and goals of the organization" (Dimond & Markowitz, 1995, p. 40). For those social work departments in hospitals that have invested time and energy in developing and maintaining strong relationships with community agencies, organizations, and the community at large (Bixby, 1995), the move to a continuum of care will be less unfamiliar and easier to accomplish.

If social workers cling to the acute care model based exclusively in the inpatient setting, many may not survive the chaos. Viewing the possibilities under a new paradigm, "the chronic complex illness model (that) assumes multiple contributing factors, with the basis of illness being biopsychosocial and the relationship among the health care systems being continuous" (Berkman, 1996, p. 543), social workers can envision and develop roles throughout the continuum of care. Shifting from an inpatient focus to assessing the needs of clients across settings, from individual care to accountability "for the health status of vulnerable at-risk populations," and from "managing a department" to managing a market for their services (Berkman, p. 548).

A NEW GAME PLAN FOR THE TEAM

The new rules imposed by managed care organizations have forced hospitals to reexamine their roles in health care. To remain competitive, hospitals have had to prove that the services they offer are superior. Many industry observers believe this creates a healthy environment, with the patient being the beneficiary of improved quality of health care services. Still, there are those who are a little more skeptical of managed care's effect on patients' well-being.

We are all familiar with the recent federal government's legislation requiring health insurance companies (many of which are managed care organizations) to allow at least 48 hours of inpatient hospital care after a vaginal birth. Before this law, there were many women leaving the hospital in as few as 6 hours after a delivery. Length of hospital stay has not just touched the labor and delivery department. The pressure to use health care resources more efficiently and effectively has resulted in patients being admitted to the hospital in a later stage of disease or illness. Patients are now being cared for as long as possible in a less resource-intensive, noninstitutional health care environment. Consequently, the patients who finally are hospitalized are more acutely ill and "their treatment involves a high level of technology care that requires counter-balancing by high touch on the part of nursing staff" (McCloskey & Grace, 1990, p. 166). Patients are also being discharged from the hospital sooner, which means they are sicker when they reenter the community.

Data show that there has been a dramatic decrease in LOS across the board under managed care. White (1995) reported LOS under managed care is 1% to 20% shorter when compared with fee-for-service LOS. The data also show that trends in the utilization of hospital services over the past decade have been characterized by a strong growth in the use of hospital outpatient services.

Although hospital reimbursement policies have contributed to the decrease in inpatient use, advances in technology have caused outpatient hospital utilization to rise rapidly. Technological advances have also significantly influenced the number of services available in hospitals that were not there just a few years ago. While moving away from providing inpatient services, many hospitals have turned their attention to providing outpatient services. Many new procedures and techniques are available in outpatient settings.

As a result of technological innovation and the growth in outpatient treatment, hospitals are offering a wider range of services to patients than in the past. Services such as rehabilitation, home health services, alcohol and chemical treatment programs, and a wide range of services and programs to meet the needs of older adults are just a few of the many outpatient services now available through many hospitals.

Utilization of nurses and social workers by the hospital has also been affected by the rising number of outpatient services now available. The objective now is to keep patients out of hospital beds. Data indicate that the percentage of nurses working in outpatient settings increased 68% between 1988 and 1992, whereas hospital inpatient nurse employment grew only 6% during the same period (Aiken, 1995).

Harrigan (1995) claimed a new skill mix will be needed so that nurse providers, previously focused on institutional-based practices, will be prepared to function in outpatient and community settings. Working as a team member in collaboration with other disciplines will be one obstacle both professions will need to overcome. One of the major challenges for educators will be modifying their educational curriculums to prepare nurses and social workers for practice in outpatient settings (see chapter 11).

CONCLUSIONS

Today, managed care organizations are placing considerable pressure on nursing to demonstrate the effect that nursing care has on the patient outcomes. According to McCloskey and Grace (1990), it is imperative that nurses be able to document the unique components of nursing care and to demonstrate that the benefits achieved with those components exceed the costs incurred in providing nursing care. To this we might add that the same is true for social workers.

It is important that both professions seize the opportunity managed care has presented to them. Now is the time that nurses and social workers can distinguish themselves and the care they give from that given by other health care providers. The future of nursing and social work will depend on the actions of nurses and social workers today.

We'll end this discussion with a note of caution. The future is filled with risks, but times of greatest risk are also times of great opportunity. Nurses and social workers must move forward, but keep in mind that the ethics of business are not always the ethics of human service professionals (Harrigan, 1995).

REFERENCES

Aiken, L. H. (1995). Transformation of the nursing workforce. *Nursing Outlook, 43,* 201–209.

Berger, C. S., Cayner, J., Jensen, G., Mizrahi, T., Scesny, A., & Trachtenberg, J. (1996). The changing scene of social work in hospitals: A report of a national study by the Society for Social Work Administrators in Health Care and NASW. *Health & Social Work, 21,* 163–173.

Berkman, B. (1996). The emerging health care world: Implications for social work practice and education. *Social Work, 41,* 541–551.

Bixby, N. B. (1995). Crisis or opportunity: A healthcare social work director's response to change. *Social Work in Health Care, 20*(4), 3–20.

Bostrom J. M. (1995). Multiple health care contracts: Changing the rules for hospital staff and systems. *Nursing Economic$, 13*(2), 99–103.

Burda, D. (1995). For-profit, not-for-profits reignite battle. *Modern Healthcare, 25*(19), 28–30.

Chamberlain, P., Chen, Y., Osuna, E., & Yamamoto, C. (1995). Innovative culture shock prescribed for health care. *Nursing Outlook, 43,* 232–234.

Dimond, M., & Markowitz, M. (1995). The effective health care social work director. *Social Work in Health Care, 20*(4), 39–59.

Fagin, C. M., & Gordon, S. (1996). The abandonment of the patient. *Nursing Outlook, 44,* 147–149.

Greene, J. (1995a). A delicate balancing act. *Modern Healthcare, 25*(11), 34–40.

Greene, J. (1995b). System hospitals earn high JCAHO marks. *Modern Healthcare, 25*(22), 33–34.

Harrigan, R. C. (1995). Health care reform: Impact of managed care on perinatal and neonatal care delivery and education. *Journal of Perinatal and Neonatal Nursing, 8*(4), 47–58.

Harrington, C., & Estes, C. L. (1994). *Health policy and nursing.* Boston: Jones and Bartlett.

Huston, C. L. (1996). Unlicensed assistive personnel: A solution to dwindling health care resources or the precursor to the apocalypse of registered nursing? *Nursing Outlook, 44*(2), 67–73.

Keepnews, D. (1996a). Nurse staffing and the problem of lack of data. *American Nurse, 28*(1), 5.

Keepnews, D. (1996b). IOM issues nurse staffing report. *American Nurse, 28*(1), 23.

Lewis, J. B. (1992). Hospital strategic management and managed care. *Topics in Healthcare Financing, 19*(2), 11–17.

Mayer, J. B. (1995). The effective healthcare social work director: Managing the social work department at Beth Israel Hospital. *Social Work in Health Care, 20*(4), 61–72.

McCloskey, J. C., & Grace H. K. (1990). *Current issues in nursing.* St. Louis, MO: Mosby.

Porter-O'Grady, T. (1994). Working with consultants on a redesign. *American Journal of Nursing, 94*(10), 33–37.

Rayburn, L. G., & Rayburn, J. M. (1996). Shift in power to hospital accountants. *Journal of Health & Social Policy, 7*(4), 23–44.

Safriet, B. J. (1992). Health care dollars and regulatory sense: The role of advanced practice nursing. *Yale Journal on Regulation, 9,* 417–487.

White, J. H. (1995). Hospitals in the new world of managed care. *Health Progress,* *76*(2), 12–16.

Wieczorek, R. R. (1996). Hospital trends—the impact on nursing practice. *Imprint,* *43*(3), 33–35.

CHAPTER 9

The Community View: New Models, New Links

Carole Wieland Pearce and Ellen Trabka

We need to practice the Willie Sutton approach to medicine. When Willie Sutton was asked why do you rob banks, he responded, 'Because that's where the money is.' In healthcare, we need to deliver services where the patients are, and the patients are at home. You break down the barriers in healthcare when you bring the services to where the patients are.—B. Grebin

Community-based nursing and social work is an old concept worth serious consideration today. First, we will visit community-based models. A brief history of community health centers begins the chapter, followed by an example of a collaborative community health center. Next, home care, school-based health care, and programs that combine hospital and community to provide care are discussed. Agencies working together in the community are the basis for the second part of the chapter. Case management in the community is discussed, followed by examples of a community nursing center; block nursing in St. Paul, Minnesota; parish nursing in Illinois; a nursing network at Carondelet St. Mary's in Tucson, Arizona; and the Community Nursing Organization pilot program that has begun at four sites across the country. These examples from across the United States provide ideas worth consideration.

COMMUNITY-BASED MODELS OF HEALTH CARE

COMMUNITY HEALTH CENTERS

Neighborhood or community health centers are not a recent innovation in health care. The history of community health centers goes back more than a century. The older community health centers in the United States are the settlement houses, established by nurses, social workers, or both in the late 19th century. There a wide variety of services was available for the neighborhood. The services might include music and art programs, adult education, courses for naturalization, public housing, and visiting nursing. The site might include a park or playground. The settlement workers coordinated the care of the neighborhood families using rudimentary case management techniques (details concerning settlement houses are in chapter 3).

In the 1920s, two centers were established in New York City: East Harlem funded by the Red Cross and Yorkville funded by the Milbank Memorial Fund. After their initial success, the city was divided into 30 health districts, and the plan was for each to have a center. Under Mayor Laguardia, seven of those centers were built with funds from the federal Public Works Administration (Alford, 1975, pp. 103–104).

Over the past 25 years, community health centers have evolved in rural and urban areas responding to Americans without availability or access to health care. Consumer input and a health-team approach are used. The funding is from a variety of federal programs or agencies, but they are staffed mostly with local providers (Hawkins & Higgins, 1993, p. 105). Often these centers have one or more professionals assigned from the National Health Service Corps (Jonas & Banta, 1986, p. 343).

The National Health Service Corps came into being in the 1970s with Rural Health Initiative money authorized by the 1970 Emergency Health Personnel Act (Pub. L. No. 91-623), which allocated resources to underdeveloped rural areas. Community health centers provided the service corps with placements for medical personnel to work in underserved areas. Currently, the National Service Corps recruits students in the health professions and provides them with scholarship money; they pay the money back by working in migrant, rural, and neighborhood health centers. The hope is that these recipients will remain in the underserved areas permanently (Sardell, 1988, pp. 111–114).

Between 1964 and 1968, under President Lyndon Johnson numerous neighborhood health centers began as part of the War on Poverty under the direction of the federal Office of Economic Opportunity (Jonas & Rosenberg, 1986, p. 146). Neighborhood health centers were designed to meet the needs of a specific community. One of the earliest was a Columbia Point housing project in the Dorchester section of Boston. The project was sponsored by Tufts University School of Medicine and underwritten initially by the Office of Economic Opportunity (Bellin & Geiger, 1976, pp. 178–180). Eventually this project developed into a comprehensive health care agency with a community focus and substantial input from the clients served there (Bellin & Geiger, 1976, pp. 199–200). Tufts also founded a rural health center in Bolivar County, Mississippi in 1966. In addition to health care, this center began a farm cooperative and organized work crews to tackle poor sanitation, rats, and an impure water supply (Klaw, 1975, p. 199). These neighborhood health centers were broader in focus than merely providing direct health care to individuals and families.

On Chicago's West Side, the Mile Square Health Center, sponsored by St. Luke's Presbyterian Hospital, was founded in 1967. This 1-mile-square area is characterized by poverty and a dense, mostly Black population. This health center was able to reach more than two thirds of the target population by the third year (Schorr, 1970, pp. 137–139). In New York City, another early center was Montefiore Neighborhood Medical Care Demonstration project in the Bronx; today it is known as the Martin Luther King Neighborhood Health Center (Hawkins & Higgins, 1993, p. 106).

By 1970 there were 49 health centers from New York to California; they operated out of a variety of settings—from new buildings to old store fronts (Schorr, 1970, p. 144). In the neighborhood health centers, an important concept was implemented: a team approach to health care. The Office of Economic Opportunity was closed in 1970 and federal support of the neighborhood health centers became the responsibility of the then Department of Health, Education, and Welfare (today the Department of Health and Human Services). With cuts in spending, these centers, now called community health centers (CHC), have become increasingly dependent on federally funded Medicare and jointly funded Medicaid (state and federal) and self pay amounts that are determined by a sliding scale (Jonas & Rosenberg, 1986, pp. 146–150).

Many CHC today have a population that includes enrollees in managed care. In a seven-site study of community health centers across the United States under managed care, Abrams, Savela, Trinity, Falik, Tutanjian, and Ulmer (1995) found that CHC were viewed as important providers in the health maintenance organization (HMO) network and compared to other providers in the network performed as well or better in the areas of cost and utilization. The arrival of managed care served as a catalyst for CHCs to improve the efficiency and capacity of their patient management techniques, financial management systems, and data systems. Those CHC with the highest percentage of enrollment in managed care, those with the greatest financial risk, or both had more primary care monitoring mechanisms and more sophisticated primary care rate negotiation than others (p. 87).

DIMOCK COMMUNITY HEALTH CENTER

The Dimock Community Health Center Early Intervention program in Boston is a model example of a program that is truly collaborative and interdisciplinary in its approach to providing specific health services.

Early Intervention (EI), sponsored by the Massachusetts Department of Public Health, is a program designed to help parents understand their children's growth and developmental needs and teach them ways in which they can help their children grow. Eligibility criteria for the program include children from birth to 3 years old who are at risk for developmental delays. This includes children born with preexisting medical problems that affect their growth and development; premature infants; children with feeding, vision, or hearing problems; developmentally challenged children; and those with behavior or attention difficulties. EI teams work together with families to formulate an Individual Family Service Plan to determine and specify which education, training, therapy, and support services the family and patient will receive. This plan may include speech, physical, and occupational therapy and pediatrician, nursing, and social work services. Additionally, developmental educators, community parents, toddler groups, parent-child groups, parent support groups, parent training and education, and referral services may be included in the plan.

The Dimock EI program provides an interdisciplinary team approach to patient care. Assessments, evaluation, and services are provided by a team of professionals and paraprofessionals from different disciplines who consult and collaborate to determine, with the family, the best approach and care plan for each individual child. In the process, traditional hierarchies normally seen within the medical establishment are broken down. Each professional and paraprofessional's skills are recognized as being equally important to the patient's treatment plan. Members of the team are often asked to substitute for one another and to cross disciplinary boundaries to learn and incorporate the skills and knowledge of other disciplines into their practices. This is termed a *transdisciplinary* approach to patient care. For example, in one case the social worker might do the medical history and in another case the community parent (CP) might take the history. The needs of the child, family, or both determine which professional or paraprofessional will do the initial assessment (Operational Standards for Early Intervention Programs in Massachusetts, 1996).

When a child is referred to EI for services, the first thing that takes place is a screening process to determine which services a child will need. The screening teams consist of varying combinations of professionals and paraprofessionals, including developmental educator, nurse, social worker, or CP. Children are screened by different teams according to their particular needs. For example, a child with medically related problems such as cerebral palsy might be screened by the nurse and the developmental educator, whereas a child with attention deficit disorder who is environmentally at risk might be screened by the social worker and a CP. An environmentally at-risk child is a child whose environment, which may include poverty, domestic violence, or substance abuse, places the child at risk for developmental delays.

Once the child is screened, a case manager is assigned to coordinate the services for the child and family. In deciding who will be the case manager, again, the needs of the client and family are considered along with the expertise of the case managers. In this particular EI program, case management is done by professionals and paraprofessionals, including social workers, nurses, occupational therapists, developmental educators, and CPs.

The CP program is a unique way to utilize paraprofessionals in providing direct health services to children and their families. In addition to being cost effective, it is also highly successful in reaching out to families who are environmentally at risk. The CP program originally started as a collaborative project between Dimock Community Health Center and Baycove Health Center 7 years ago and was funded by grant money. The pilot project ended 2 years ago and has been refunded.

The CP program was envisioned as a support service for parents with environmentally at-risk children. The role of CPs is to provide a full range of services to parents and families and to function as role models and change advocates in the larger health care delivery system. Community parents can be involved in all aspects of the EI service delivery program. By collaborating with the EI professional, the CP can participate in case management services and in team evaluations; provide direct service through home visits; and serve as a staff member on various groups such as parent support groups, parent-child groups, and child-focused groups (Standard Service Contract for the Community Moms Project, 1995).

Community parents are chosen for the job based on their qualifications as parents who are active and known in the community and who enjoy working with children. They must be residents of the community and have experience raising children. Their personal characteristics must include warmth, empathy, sensitivity, maturity, and openness. Education requirements include a high school diploma or a GED (General Education Degree) (Standard Service Contract for the Community Moms Project, 1995).

Training of the CP is done on the job through a series of workshops, observations, and practice in group activities. CPs receive an intensive 2- to 3-week training on child development and assessment procedures, including social-emotional and speech and language assessments. They are trained by a supervisor to do home visits and full case management. They coordinate yearly assessments of clients, coordinate discharge planning, and participate in partial or complete evaluations.

One of the most important functions of a CP is to advocate for parents and families. Because parents do not see them as another social worker, CPs are able to develop relationships with the parents quicker. It is less scary for some parents to deal with a CP than with a social worker. The CPs' unique perspectives as parents and as members of the community enable them to be able to relate to the experiences of the parents.

CPs advocate for families in many ways. For example, CPs help families get the services they need in the community. This might entail accompanying a parent to housing court to receive housing or helping them find a shelter if they are homeless. Another way in which the CPs advocate for families is by connecting families who have already gone through the evaluation process with families whose children are anticipating an evaluation. Because evaluation is a difficult process for parents to undergo, it is helpful for families to share experiences and support each other. Community parents also help to translate clinical language to parents so that they can better understand the evaluation.

One of the CPs at the Dimock Health Center speaks Spanish and English. Part of her job is to act as a bridge between the two cultures. Many Latino families are unfamiliar with the working of the United States health and human service system. The CP helps those families navigate through the system and provides translation services.

One of the CPs is certified as a perinatal outreach worker and family support assistant. This role encompasses teaching parenting skills, dealing with environmental issues such as substance abuse, providing education concerning its effects on children, and talking with and supporting parents through their detoxification programs. The role also includes providing anticipatory guidance for parents on childcare issues and discussing everyday issues. This service is especially helpful for postpartum mothers who are environmentally at risk.

HOME CARE

Home care has changed dramatically since managed care arrived. Sending hospitalized patients home earlier than in the past has led to health care delivery in the home that one would have only dreamed of 10 years ago. Full service home care companies are able to provide a complete array of home services (Lumsdon, 1994, p. 46). These home care companies are able to provide cost savings to those they contract with, mostly managed care companies.

Home infusion and respiratory therapies have led the way (Lumsdon, 1994, p. 46). There are dramatic examples of care in the home. Home Technology Health Care in Nashville, Tennessee delivers home care for pregnant women who develop diabetes instead of the usual hospitalization for tests, assessment, and education. It costs about 15% of the price of hospitalization. They also care for stabilized low-birth-weight babies who are sent home in isolettes, cutting the cost in half (Lumsdon, 1994, p. 46). Abbey Healthcare Group Inc. of Costa Mesa, California works with people who have the top 20 disabilities that cost employers 80% of their health care dollars, such as cardiology, diabetes, respiratory problems, and pregnancy (Lumsdon, 1994, p. 46).

A Home Care Program for Children

In New York City, St. Mary's Home Care Program serves children in all five boroughs. This home care program for children began in the late 1970s. They adapted the "nursing home without walls" concept and convinced the New York State Department of Health to accept the fact that children with complex medical needs are more appropriately and economically cared for at home (Grebin, 1994, p. 5).

SCHOOL-BASED PROGRAMS

Robert Wood Johnson Foundation

The Robert Wood Johnson Foundation appropriated nearly $5 million for demonstration projects in 69 schools in Utah, North Dakota, New York, and Colorado in 1978. The granting of this money was based on programs in Cambridge, Massachusetts, Posen-Robbins, Illinois, and Galveston, Texas (Meeker, DeAngelis, Berman, Freeman, & Oda, 1986, p. 87). The three programs were very different and will be very briefly described.

The Cambridge program provided for most of the children's medical care using nurse practitioners. The outreach clinics were located in the schools and were able to provide convenient and timely health care for school-aged children, thereby reducing the use of the emergency room considerably and providing overall savings to the community. Screening and other population-based services were limited (Meeker et al., 1986, p. 87).

The Posen–Robbins program specifically targeted families on Medicaid and aimed to provide access to care for them. The program at Posen–Robbins (a suburb of Chicago) provided primary care and did not emphasize the other services needed by the community such as screening, immunization surveillance, and education. They provide services to a large number of children but have not become financially self-sufficient as they had hoped (Meeker et al., 1986, p. 87).

The Galveston program never aimed to provide direct care, but instead provided preventive and educational services with little primary care. The emphasis was on detection of health problems at the school-based clinics and referral of children to community providers who were usually at the medical school (Meeker et al., 1986, p. 87).

SCHOOL-BASED TEEN PARENT PROGRAM

In Wisconsin, teen pregnancy programs began in 1973 when the state legislature provided special educational money to fund programs for teen parents. In the beginning, the school-based programs served only females and offered remedial academic subjects. Today, the services still include basic skills for academic subjects, but also include social services resources; information on available counseling; vocational guidance, career development, and employment education; resources for maternal and child health and related education. These programs use social workers as case managers and have become very comprehensive; they now include the school-age fathers (Davis, 1992, pp. 27–29).

PRIVATE CASE MANAGEMENT

One of the first private geriatric practices, the Aging Network Services of Bethesda, Maryland, was founded in 1982. This agency, staffed by professional social workers with a Master of Social Work degree, provides services specifically designed for elders and their families. This service is needed in this age of elderly persons living alone while their children often live geographically distant. The agency has established an extensive network of colleagues throughout the country to serve families and is capable of providing services in most metropolitan areas and select outlying areas. The staff serve as therapists, service brokers, and supervisors of social workers with less education. An extensive assessment is made of the individual and family plus the environment of the elderly person. Assessment is ongoing over the time of the service (Lebow & Kane, 1992, pp. 37–39).

HOSPITAL AND COMMUNITY-BASED PROGRAMS

TREATMENT-TEAM MODEL

Olson, Rickles, and Travlik discussed a treatment-team model of case management that provides care both in the hospital and in the community. The Waltham-Weston Hospital, a community hospital near Boston, has developed a team approach to managing patients with psychiatric illnesses. This service, unlike most case management, is available for all patients, not just those who have chronic illnesses (1995, p. 254). The treatment team managed care agent is involved directly with the patient on a clinical basis (p. 255). In this model of care, any patient who needs more intense mental health care is seen by a licensed health care professional, called the *managed care clinician*, at the hospital. The managed care clinician acts as the managed care agent and becomes part of the clinical treatment team. The managed care clinician consults with the primary therapist and makes a decision concerning the level of care needed. The clinician considers more intensive treatment and makes arrangements if needed. A direct encounter may enable a patient to feel the crisis has been addressed and avoid hospitalization. Referrals can be made to a service that is part of the team. Because of the team approach, the response is as therapeutic as possible, and transitions between levels of care are coordinated between team members. Medications can begin immediately along with admission to a partial hospitalization and individual, group therapy, or both. Patients deemed self-destructive can be admitted overnight for observation and then followed by the managed care agent until they enter a partial hospitalization program (pp. 253–254). This model of managed care meets the criteria for health care today: high quality and cost effective with all decisions made by a team (p. 255).

LOS ANGELES PEDIATRIC AIDS NETWORK

A comprehensive care system for children with HIV and their families, known as the Los Angeles Pediatric AIDS Network (LAPAN) is funded under the Title V program that provides health care for children with chronic illnesses. The program began in 1988 and was sponsored by California Children Services. The program is headquartered at Children's Hospital Los Angeles; social work case managers are at each site. The children receive care at one of seven hospitals (one public-state, three public-county, three private nonprofit), with additional community-based organizations providing other support services. The services include case management, community education, service coordination, and a resource bank. The planning for these families includes a culturally sensitive approach and support in their daily activities. Careful planning for the safe education of these children is necessary; support groups for parents may be very helpful (Kaplan, 1992, pp. 77–83).

AGENCIES WORKING TOGETHER IN THE COMMUNITY: NEW MODELS, NEW ALLIANCES

In the 1980s and early 1990s, a number of innovative programs began throughout the United States. In the Midwest, block nursing and modern parish nursing have their origins; in the Southwest, Carondelet St. Mary's has developed a nursing network. In 1994, four Community Nursing Organizations began a Medicare demonstration project. All of these programs have case management as the cornerstone. These example all have one thing in common; they use professional nurses as case managers. In Wisconsin, social workers are case managers in a comprehensive teenage pregnancy program that includes outreach, academic education, pregnancy and parenting education, vocational guidance and career development (Davis, 1992, pp. 27–29). They are also case managers in early intervention programs for disabled infants and toddlers across the country (Hare & Clark, 1992, pp. 51–74). In Massachusetts a visiting nurses association uses nurses and social workers serving as dual case managers.

CASE MANAGEMENT IN THE COMMUNITY SETTING

Case management can be either institutional or community based (Kelly & Maas, 1994, p. 136). Community based nurse case managers assist patients in developing greater self-care abilities and in assuming more responsibility for their health care (Kelly & Maas, 1994, p. 172).

> In providing services to patients and their families, nurse case managers may evaluate health status, screen for common health problems, teach self-reliance and monitoring, obtain community-based support, coordinate access to needed health services, facilitate short- and long-term planning for health management, make referrals to other health care providers, manage nursing care, coordinate other care, broker services, serve as a primary provider, and/or assist patients to negotiate the health care system. (Kelly & Maas, 1994, p. 173)

Services provided elsewhere in the system are not duplicated (Kelly & Maas, 1994, p. 173).

Case management in the community setting is often employed when patients need social or medical intervention over time because of chronic conditions such as AIDS and severe mental illness. These people have a variety of health care, social service, and psychological needs. Case management can include intake and assessment, planning for services, making referrals and system linkages, monitoring services received and status of clients (Mor, Piette, & Fleishman, 1989, p. 139), and advocacy. Linking clients with appropriate community-based services and rationing expensive inpatient care services decreases the total cost of care (Mor et al., 1989, p. 139). Whether these goals can be realized is unclear.

In a randomized clinical trial of patients who are severely mentally ill who were handled by case management, the treatment group did not demonstrate significant improvement in satisfaction with their lives or psychosocial adjustment with case management. A shift from 24-hour and emergency care to outpatient services did occur, but the cost actually increased slightly (Jerrell & Hu, 1989, p. 233).

Case management can also be employed in posthospital management of frail older people. Evaluators of the Robert Wood Johnson Program for Hospital Initiatives in Long-Term Care found that case management was seen as an adjunct to adequate medical care. It was also seen as a combination of a way the hospital met its mission of community service and a tool to attract new customers. Case management has the potential to modify the boundaries of the hospital's role in long-term care. Most experimental programs were unable to document a change in outcomes as a result of case management (MacAdam et al., 1989, pp. 743–744), and some actually proved to be more expensive (Capitman, Haskins, & Bernstein, 1986, p. 403). Those programs that were least expensive featured targeting of costs and mechanisms for identification of clients (Capitman et al., 1986, p. 403).

COMMUNITY NURSING CENTER

Abbottsford Community Health Center in Philadelphia was one of the original seven Section 340a health centers created by the Disadvantaged Minority Health Improvement Act of 1990 (Pub. L. No. 101-527) and funded by the U.S. Department of Health and Human Services. This program was specifically aimed at improving access for public housing residents to comprehensive primary and preventive health care. Abbottsford was the only center managed by a nurse practitioner (Jenkins & Torrisi, 1995, p. 119).

The nurse practitioners at the center have contracted with two publicly funded HMOs to provide primary care for the residents of public housing, who are almost exclusively Black. Data for the first 12 months revealed that the family nurse practitioners' (FNP) patients used the emergency department 43% as often and had only 38% of the in-hospital days as the Medicaid patients handled by the family physicians in the same HMO. The FNP also had 1.8 more encounters than the HMO as aggregate, and total annual cost was $56.72 versus $97.96 for the aggregate (Jenkins & Torrisi, 1995, p. 119).

The FNPs, who are case managers, deliver care on a continuum and integrate services inside and outside the organization. The primary care services at the community nursing center include individual counseling and mental health treatment by a psychologist; prenatal and diabetic education by two community health nurses; van transportation to the pharmacy and specialists; outreach and advocacy by five resident outreach workers who also run a variety of support groups for all ages; education, support, advocacy, and peer education by community resident leaders; and consultation by internist, pediatrician, and perinatologist. The FNPs independently refer patients to a specialist or for hospitalization and order radiology and laboratory tests (Jenkins & Torrisi, 1995, pp. 119–120).

BLOCK NURSING

Many nursing home residents actually can remain in their homes if appropriate services are available. Five percent of our elderly population are in nursing homes (Eustis, 1984, p. 58). Many of them could be managed at home if they were able to obtain help there. Of those who need some type of assistance, it is estimated that between 55% and 58% are cared for informally by their families, friends, and neighbors (Eustis, 1984, p. 32).

The Living at Home/Block Nurse Program (LAH/BNP) began in 1982 in a public health district called St. Anthony Park, in St. Paul, Minnesota. The program was designed to keep the 30% who can to stay in their homes, thereby providing the services they need (Jamieson, 1996, p. 22). Many of the original participants were nurses and social workers (Jamieson & Martinson, 1983, p. 270).

This community program uses Medicare reimbursement; alternative funding; sliding scale personal payments; professionals and volunteers in the community, plus an informal network of family, neighbors, friends, and service clubs, such as Rotary Club and the Boy Scouts (Jamieson, 1990, p. 250; Jamieson & Martinson, 1983, p. 270), to provide information, care management-service coordination, social and support services, nursing, and other needed services (Jamieson, 1996, p. 22).

The program's goal is to enhance the family's ability to meet their relative's needs. Block nurses, block companions, and block volunteers provide services to their neighbors who are age 65 or older. The block nurses assess the clients and families and provide nursing care. The nurses serve as gatekeepers to ensure that only necessary services are provided, and that quality care is delivered. Block volunteers are trained paraprofessionals who provide homemaker and home health aide services; their training is at the local vocational-technical institute. Block volunteers are neighbors trained to counsel and emotionally support their peers (Jamieson, 1987, p . 1227). Social workers supervise the counseling, but the block nurses are the care coordinators (case managers) (Jamieson & Martinson, 1983, p. 273).

Participants, paid workers, and volunteers all live within the community. Existing city, county, state, and private agencies and available resources are used, negating the need for anything new or a layer of bureaucracy. Paid workers are employees of an existing public health agency with mechanisms for client's charts, payroll, access to third-party payers, and quality assurance programs already in place (Jamieson, 1990, p. 252). This program has grown from one pilot community (St. Anthony Park) lasting 7 years, to three replication sites (Highland Park, North End-South Como, and Atwater) for 3 years, to fifteen programs in Minnesota. In 1995, a national demonstration program was scheduled to begin (Jamieson, 1990, p. 253; Jamieson, 1996, p. 22). The block nurse approach can be a step in the development of a community nursing network that keeps the chronically ill out of hospitals and nursing homes (Martinson, Jamieson, O'Grady, & Sime, 1985, p. 29).

This is one of the few community programs that actually demonstrates clearly that keeping the elderly at home in the community saves money. An external evaluator examined the 3-year three-site replication program and estimated 38% of those served would have been in nursing homes. The program costs less than $500 a month for each of the participants to live at home, where they want to be, compared with approximately $2,000 a month in a nursing home (Jamieson, 1996, p. 22).

Early trends from the LAH/BNP were (a) 80% of the referrals were word of mouth; (b) a neighborhood participation project seems to be more successful than a superimposed system; (c) the community adapts programs to meet its need without the usual bureaucratic constraints; (d) the community has become sensitive to the needs of the elderly persons in the community and asks for group projects; (e) and neighbors report quality control information informally to the staff who live in the community. Families and neighbors have become more involved, and the family is more able to meet the needs of the elderly person. Approximately 15% of the participants have chosen to be discharged from a nursing home to block nurse care. People plan for their retirement differently when they know services will be available at home, and some have chosen to die at home using this type of care. It is estimated that 25% of hospitalizations were prevented through health education, early intervention, and prevention. Care management takes less time because staff members know the participants and their support system. Combining homemaker and home health aide functions into one job is more efficient, and staff is available at odd hours and during inclement weather. Even after a case is closed, workers and volunteers often maintain informal contact; this addresses the issue of prevention (Jamieson, 1990, p. 253).

Jamieson (1996) clearly pointed out that this program is *community based* (by and with the people) as opposed to *community oriented* (to and for people). Many citizens are involved here, not just a few. Some of the professionals and volunteers become lasting friends with the participants. LAH/BNP connects with agencies and organizations for services and creates new ones where they're not available (p. 22). The program was designed by six persons; four were nurses. Their goals were case management and changing the long-term care delivery system. They believed that people banding together can change the system and have the power to change government through election of officials. The message was change and hope (p. 24).

In this program, as with others discussed here, case management is needed to coordinate the fragmented health and long-term care system. LAH/BNP prefers the term *care management* to *case management* (Jamieson, 1996, p. 22). Why not use *health care management* or even *health management* instead of case management? Included in their care is diagnosis and management of acute episodes and management of disabilities and chronic illness, activity-in-daily-living deficits, social isolation, and failing mental capacity. In the center of the care plan are the participant and the family; the block nurse is the person advocating, arranging, coordinating, and delivering services. The block nurse holds weekly care conferences in the community, often with the volunteers, where non-nursing support is integrated. Some examples are the Rotary Club repairing fallen plaster and cleaning gutters, Boy Scouts painting, community members providing meals on weekends and holidays and writing letters and Christmas cards, free delivery by the local grocery store, and transportation to church. Participants often receive these services before they need nursing care. Fund raising is necessary to cover services entitlements don't cover (Jamieson, 1996, pp. 22–23).

PARISH NURSING

Often overlooked when considering community-based nursing is the local congregation or place of worship and parish nursing. "What particularly distinguishes parish nursing is how it keeps body and soul together by clearly linking personal faith and health" (Martin, 1996, p. 25). The population served by this community-based nursing is the community of faith (Djupe, 1996, pp. 140–141). Miller (1995) stated "The broad concept of spirituality is central to many religious belief systems" (p. 258). In the administration of medical care, the spiritual aspect of the lives of those we care for is too often ignored or treated as the peripheral demographic characteristic.

Granger Westbert, a retired Lutheran chaplain, is generally credited with developing holistic health centers in churches in the 1960s, which evolved into parish nursing in the 1980s (King, Lakin, & Striepe, 1993, p. 27). Actually, parish nursing has a long history in Europe, New Zealand, and Australia (Simington, Olson, & Douglass, 1996, p. 20). The first institutionally based paid parish nurse program in the United States was initiated by the Lutheran General Health System in Illinois in 1984. Four protestant and two Roman Catholic congregations formed a partnership; the Lutheran General System funded the parish nurse and educational program while the congregation and institution shared the salary cost. In 1988, Trinity Medical Center (formerly United Medical Center) in western Illinois began a sister program. In 10 years, the two programs have grown and now serve more than 80,000 congregational members of 13 denominations. The 53 parish nurses serve 59 rural, suburban, and inner city congregations (Djupe, 1996, p. 142). In 1992 there were 1,500 parish nurses (King et al., 1993, p. 27).

The church is unique in that people turn to the church at special times in life such as birth, baptism, confirmation, marriage, and death. There is a certain continuity in peoples' lives around the church, and the congregation consists of people of all ages. The parish nurse is the anchor for individuals and families as they have contact with community agencies. They cannot work alone, but need a corps of volunteers to carry out this work (Djupe, 1996, p. 145).

King and others compare parish nursing to public health nursing (1993, p. 29). The population of interest is the congregation and attention is directed toward subgroups (aggregates in public health language) within the church such as youth, older members, and single parents. Miskelly (1995) conducted a community needs assessment of an urban southern Wisconsin church using a self-developed wellness and needs assessment survey that identified the demographics, risks, medical conditions, and the most popular educational and support group choices. From these findings a parish nursing program could be planned for the population of any specific congregation.

Parish nurses provide services such as personal health counseling, health education, organizing and supporting volunteers, resources and referrals, and interpreting the connection between faith and health. The services may be provided in the community, home, church, nursing home, or on the telephone.

The place of worship is an important health resource, especially for the poor and underserved. The parish nurse, as member of a pastoral team, integrates the resources of the individual, community, and health care. These nurses collaborate with school nurses, home health nurses, and nurses in Medicare settings. Typically, they do not carry out medical procedures or medical functions (Djupe, 1996, pp. 140–141); they do not duplicate existing services (Drummond, Buss, & Ladigo, 1992, p. 20; Simington et al., 1996, p. 22). They are able to maintain long-term relationships with those they care for (Djupe, 1996, pp. 140–141).

Parish nursing models vary. The implementation might be administered by a hospital or community health center; an individual church; regional diocese, synod, or board; or a coalition among churches of different denominations, health institutions, social organizations, and educational institutions (Simington et al., 1996, pp. 21–22). The parish nurse may be employed by a church or parish (Dunkle, 1996), a hospital (Drummond et al., 1992, p. 20) or community health center (Dunkle, 1996, p. 55; Simington et al., 1996, p. 21), or work as a volunteer (Dunkle, 1996, p. 55); most work part time. Those who are volunteers often receive money for supplies, gas, and continuing education (Dunkle, 1996, p. 55). Funding can be a continuing struggle for many parish nurses (Schank, Weis, & Matheus, 1996, p. 13). Often the parish nurse reports to a health or oversight committee.

Parish nurses give personal counseling (Djupe, 1996, pp. 142–144; Schank et al., 1996, p. 12). They discuss personal problems; make home, nursing home, and hospital visits; and recommend medical intervention when necessary. The issues often dealt with are parenting, dealing with teenagers, relationships with spouses or other family members, and aging parents. End-of-life decisions can be discussed with the pastor and nurse within the context of values and faith (Djupe, 1996, pp. 142–144). Support group organization enhances the healing and caring community of the church (King et al., 1993, p. 28).

The social worker could have a collaborative role in this community-based health care; the social worker's skills lend themselves to many of the roles of the parish nurse. Social workers could be invaluable in the counseling role and also in intervening with families, significant others, and groups, as they excel in this expertise. They also are very knowledgeable about available services and can provide these resources readily.

Much of the parish nurse's time is spent educating the parishioners (Djupe, 1996, pp. 142–144; Dunkle, 1996, p. 56; King et al., 1993, p. 27; Schank et al., 1996, p. 12). The role may include reviewing discharge instructions or the side effects of a medication or explaining a diagnostic test or procedure. Preventive care is taught concerning, for example, skin cancer or reducing cardiovascular risk. The education is provided one on one, in groups (Dunkle, 1996, p. 56), seminars, newsletters, articles or columns in church bulletins, and bulletin boards. Support groups may be facilitated over such issues as weight loss, care giving, and parenting (Djupe, 1996, pp. 142–144). Health screening may also be provided (Simington et al., 1996, p. 23).

The parish nurse advocates for the parishioners (Djupe, 1996, pp. 142–144; Dunkle, 1996, p. 56; King et al., 1993, p. 27; Schank et al., 1996, p. 12) with health-related resources, the congregation, and the community. Included may be self-help; physician care; community, state, or federal agencies; housing, shelters, food pantries, retirement facilities, and nursing homes; hospitals; home care; elder care; psychotherapists; and legal and financial counselors (Djupe, 1996, pp. 142–144). Troubleshooting helps prevent parishioners from getting lost in the system; it may mean perhaps loaning out and teaching proper use of crutches or a wheelchair or discovering ineffective medications are outdated (Dunkle, 1996, p. 56).

Many churches have a volunteer structure in place. The parish nurse selects and trains the members to be volunteers (Dunkle, 1996, p. 56; Simington et al., 1996, p. 22) and is the volunteer coordinator (Dunkle, 1996, p. 56). The parish nurse is a clinical resource and supports the volunteers and aids them in broadening and extending the help available within the congregation (Djupe, 1996, pp. 142–144).

Parish nurses carry out this specialized work because it offers a unique opportunity to counsel with individuals and families about the deeper beliefs and values that affect their health. This is accomplished along with health committees, a pastoral team, and lay leaders (Djupe, 1996, pp. 142–144). Shared responsibilities and collaborative efforts among community health care providers enhance effective health promotion and improve healthcare services (King et al., 1993, p. 31). Why not have a social worker included and collaborating with them as well? The work they do is similar to case management. A majority of their time is spent with older church members; the primary concerns are loneliness, isolation, relationships, access to services, grief and loss, questions related to a certain illness, and hospitalization (Djupe, 1996, pp. 142–144). It has been a common model, at least in New England, to have a social services committee in churches and to even have a social worker on the staff paid for by the congregation (Old South Church in Boston and others had a paid social worker on staff).

Parish nurses who work in the inner city have additional issues that are important; those issues are rooted in poverty and crime. Resources are scarce; violence and drugs are common; and parishioners are at risk for social isolation, poor health, injury, and death. Basic needs such as food, clothing, housing, and heat may be the most pressing issues. Health issues must be considered part of the social context. Parishioners may fear leaving their homes. Homelessness has led to churches providing shelter and meals (Djupe, 1996, pp. 144–145).

The Parish Nursing Services at Lutheran General Health Systems have developed partnerships between a large health care system and congregations and have moved toward working with clients as partners. They, too, have learned some lessons. All persons, even the homeless and mentally ill, search for God and for meaning in their lives. You cannot give up on people and must be committed to long-term relationships. Each person may have a different ability to be responsible. For those who have little trust, building relationships takes a very long time. What persons believe they need is very important and they must be consulted. Parish nurses cannot act on suppositions and prejudices. One must recognize the need to let go. Group support of the parish nurses occurs at bimonthly group meeting that are held for education, support, and sharing cases (Djupe, 1996, pp. 146–147).

Parish nursing is an opportunity for nurses and social workers to practice autonomously and implement population-based appropriate wellness programs. We must seize this opportunity to develop, implement, and evaluate community programs that advance community wellness (Miskelly, 1995, p. 13).

A NURSING NETWORK: CARONDELET ST. MARY'S NURSING ENTERPRISE

In an attempt to enhance professional nurse accountability at Carondelet St. Mary's hospital in Tucson, Arizona, patients were charged for nursing services. Unexpectedly, the result was that nursing became a business as well as a service, and the scope of nursing expanded beyond the hospital walls. When they began charging people for nursing services, health care was making the early transition from reimbursement to prospective payment. There was an increasing need to create links between nurses inside the hospital and to beyond the hospital walls to help people manage their health care because of the continued need for care after hospitalization. Eventually the nursing network encompassing all aspects of nursing in the community and the hospital became a reality. Incidentally, in 1992, nursing was the largest contributor to St. Mary's profit margin (Michaels, 1992, p. 77).

The nursing enterprise created at St. Mary's was based on a vision, not strategic planning. Nursing case management was the vehicle by which they expanded their impact on recovery from illness. People were helped to complete their convalescence, improve their self-care skills, and receive support when self-care was not sufficient. To manage these clients across the spectrum of care, they shifted the emphasis from illness to health and developed nurse-managed community health centers. People who did not need nurse case management could receive education, guidance for health maintenance, disease prevention, and health promotion (Michaels, 1992, pp. 77–78).

Nursing began contracting with payors and making contracts to provide a variety of services: establishing a health center at a life-care residence, nurse case management for substance-abusing pregnant women enrolled in an HMO for the medically indigent, and case management of medical-surgical patients with multiple hospitalizations. St. Mary's also established a nursing HMO for case management and nursing services in the community for handling health issues for the 5% of the older population who are enrolled in an HMO and are at highest risk (Michaels, 1992, p. 78).

The nursing network at Carondelet St. Mary's is composed of nurses in complimentary roles with St. Mary's Hospital and Health Center and the Carondelet Corporation, which consists of nurses in the hospital, nursing home, hospice, home health, and community health center. At the hub of this network is the nurse case manager.

COMMUNITY NURSE CASE MANAGEMENT AT CARONDELET ST. MARY'S

Nurse case management at the Carondelet St. Mary's Hospital and Health Center was designed to improve the quality of care and maximize accessibility, while being cost effective. The nurse case managers develop collaborative relationships with their patients. The patients' choices concerning heath care are understood and honored, and they are helped to recognize patterns in their choices and the connection to outcomes. The patient is viewed holistically; many case managers attribute this to traditional Indian medicine that connects the spiritual aspect of a person with the environment and all other aspects. Nurse case managers offer a more comprehensive assessment of health than other professionals who serve as case managers due to the combination of direct nursing care and case management (Newman, Lamb, & Michaels, 1991, p. 405).

At Carondelet St. Mary's, the nursing network, with the professional nurse case manager (PNCM) at the center, enables patients to access care that includes nursing services in the community, hospice, long-term or skilled care, rehabilitation, education, home health, and ambulatory and acute care (Ethridge, 1991, p. 22). Patients are followed throughout the nursing network by the case manager (Ethridge & Lamb, 1989, p. 31). Nurse case managers carry a caseload of approximately 40 patients (30 in the community and 10 in the acute care setting). Additionally, the case manager has 40 to 50 stabilized patients whose ongoing evaluation is a monthly phone call (Ethridge & Lamb, 1989, p. 30).

The nurse case manager in partnership with the patient coordinates services for self-care and negotiates support services when needed. Patients are most often referred during an inpatient admission, but can enter the system from any part of the continuum and from other community organizations, social services, physicians, or payors (Kelly & Maas, 1994, p. 172). The case manager screens the patients to determine their suitability for nurse case management (Ethridge, 1991, p. 24). The two primary reasons patients are admitted into case management are that they have a chronic illness and are at risk, and they need temporary services for recovery from an acute episode (Kelly & Maas, 1994, p. 172).

A nurse case manager is assigned to patients when they enter the program. In the community the nurse case manager makes home visits or telephones patients; coordinates, negotiates, evaluates, and modifies the care and services as needed; and makes referrals to physicians, acute care services, and nursing centers in a timely manner. The intensity of the services reflects individual patient need and is evaluated and modified to meet changing needs. Patients are placed on inactive status, discharged, or transferred to another care giver when case management services are no longer needed. If a patient managed in the community is admitted to the hospital, the case manager works with the hospital staff for continuity of care and to develop or confirm the discharge plans (Kelly & Maas, 1993, p. 172).

Nursing case management for Carondelet St. Mary's has met the goals of preventing admissions and breaking the readmission cycle. When a person is admitted to acute care, nurse case management works to reduce the length of stay; intervention at a lower level of acuity results in less emergency department use, a decrease in critical care, and cost savings (Ethridge & Lamb, 1989, p. 32). The result is improved health status, enhanced patient satisfaction, and more appropriate use of resources (Kelly & Maas, 1994, p. 173).

Lamb and Stempel (1994) in their qualitative study of 16 participants with 13 case managers, examined the process of case management instead of the outcomes. They found that individuals grow into an insider expert. This process consists of three intrapersonal and interpersonal phases that build on each other: bonding, working, and changing (p. 9). "Bonding is a series of experiences during which the client and family come to believe that the nurse case manager has the expertise to help them manage their medical problems and will be responsive to their needs" (p. 9). During the working phase the patient begins to identify behaviors, attitudes, and reactions that may have interfered with the ability to use the health care system effectively and led to an exacerbation of the illness (p. 9). Many develop the feeling of a sense of mastery over their illness and are willing to try new behaviors because the nurse case manager is there for them (pp. 10–11). During the third phase, clients experience behavior changes such as lifestyle alterations, recognition of the early signs of exacerbation of a chronic illness, and seeking care earlier. Many doubted they would have attempted changes without the support of the nurse case manager (p. 11).

COMMUNITY HEALTH CENTERS

Carondelet St. Mary's has a system of 14 community-based clinics where nurse practitioners provide health screening, health promotion, and counseling services. The centers are most often used by those who are healthier than those seen by PNCM. The people tend to be poor and elderly. The community health centers are located where their clientele have easy access: low-income housing projects, mobile home parks, and retirement communities. St. Mary's financially supports all the centers except for one retirement community where the rent covers the cost (Michaels, 1992, pp. 80–81).

The centers are staffed by adult nurse practitioners who focus on health risk appraisal, health promotion, and strategies for lifestyle changes. Screening is available for blood pressure, cholesterol, and blood sugar; counseling is available for special diets, nutrition, stress reduction, medications, exercise, and community resources. These are places where, in a nonrushed environment, people can sit and talk about their health concerns and develop a partnership with the nurse practitioners (Michaels, 1992, p. 81).

The community centers depend on the community for support and volunteers; space and some equipment are provided by the community.

Residents at each site set up the center, greet clients, and aid them in access to services. A pattern of neighbor-to-neighbor referral has occurred as they become an integral part of the community. Seasonal visitors make up almost half of the visitors, and 39% have no physician in Tucson (Michaels, 1992, p. 81).

Because of the community health centers, early identification and treatment of common health problems among elderly and poor clients, such as hypertension, diabetes, and depression, have occurred. There is a high level of customer satisfaction, and people state they are able to care for themselves better (Michaels, 1992, p. 81).

Nursing HMO

In 1990, Carondelet St. Mary's began a nursing HMO. Both the PNCM and the community nursing services were offered to a medical HMO to complement their medical services and emphasize nursing's contribution. From a business viewpoint, St. Mary's believed managed care was coming, and that a nursing HMO would strengthen the business opportunities for the organization and PNCM and for nursing (Michaels, 1992, p. 82).

A nursing HMO was created and a capitated contract was negotiated to provide the medical HMO with nurse case management and community nursing services for 5% of their highest risk enrollees at a per-person per-month rate. The services are aimed at recovery from illness and maintaining health. Due to capitation, Medicare limits on services did not apply and a wider range of nursing services is offered. Those at highest risk are identified and assisted both inside and outside the hospital (Michaels, 1992, p. 82).

If the person is homebound and requires skilled nursing care, the Medicare home health nurse provides the care. The most common referrals to Medicare home health service are those learning insulin self-administration or wound care or those in need of rehabilitation at home (Michaels, 1992, p. 82).

PNCM serves as the primary provider in the community for those who do not meet Medicare home health criteria. The PNCM may secure the services of a licensed provider, skilled home health aide, companion, or homemaker. Commonly, the person needing services has just been discharged from a skilled nursing facility or hospital and is at high risk for crisis and readmission if not assisted to return to self-care (Michaels, 1992, p. 82).

The PNCMs work mostly in the community but do make hospital visits. Other PNCMs (outside the HMO) screen hospitalized patients for high risk potential and track their self-care ability throughout the hospitalization, stay at a skilled nursing facility, or both. Outcomes like self-care status, well-being, and empowerment were translated into broader health care outcomes. By comparing hospital discharges, days in the hospital, and emergency visits before and after the HMO started, they found during the first 5 months a savings of $800,000 for the medical HMO (Michaels, 1992, pp. 83–84).

COMMUNITY NURSING ORGANIZATION

The most recent innovation is the Community Nursing Organization (CNO) demonstration project. Two of the sites have already been discussed in detail: block nursing in St. Paul and Carondelet St. Mary's nursing network in Tucson. Early in 1994, four CNOs began functioning as a Medicare demonstration project. The sites are the Visiting Nurse Service in New York City; the LAH/BNP in St. Paul, Minnesota; Carle Clinic Association in Urbana, Illinois; and Carondelet Health Care in Tucson, Arizona. The sites vary greatly in organizational structure, geography, and cultural populations. The Visiting Nurse Service is the oldest nonprofit home health agency in the country. The professional nurses in the LAH/BNP grassroots community delivery system work in their own local communities. Carle Clinic Association serves a rural population and is one of the largest physician group practices in the country. Carondelet is part of a very large multihospital system serving rural and urban populations with a large Hispanic population (Lamb, 1995, pp. 18–19).

The 3-year demonstration, funded by the Health Care Financing Agency, has the goals of improving the quality of ambulatory and community care for persons receiving Medicare and promoting efficient and timely use of community services covered by Medicare guidelines. A capitation method similar to an HMO's is used for funding; CNOs receive a monthly payment according to a formula based on gender, age, activities-of-daily-living indicators, and use of home health service within the past 6 months (Lamb, 1995, pp. 18–19).

The CNO model offers professional nursing care in community and neighborhood settings; the eligibility criteria are not rigid. Registered nurses are available to assist demonstration participants to manage their health care needs (Lamb, 1995, pp. 18–19). Each site must provide mandated services to the CNO enrollees: nurse case management; home health care that includes skilled nursing, social work, home health aides, and physical, occupational, and speech therapy; outpatient physical therapy and speech therapy, and short-term behavioral management; medical equipment and supplies; ambulance services for emergency and nonemergency care; and some prosthetics (Lamb, 1995, p. 20).

> The participating nurses share the mission of the demonstration project: To create a nurse-managed delivery system that seeks to assure the quality, access, and affordable services for Medicare beneficiaries. This system sets forth a new structure for the delivery of selected community and ambulatory services and incorporates strategies to maximize continuity, care coordination, and active consumer participation. The Community Nursing Organization model provides an effective infrastructure for building consumer-oriented and cost-effective managed care networks. (Lamb, 1995, p. 19)

Lessons have been learned from the project at the Carondelet site. It is a major challenge to enroll sufficient members to meet budget demands. Those who do enroll, do so because they wish to stay healthy. Consumers need to be educated concerning exactly what a CNO is and what it is not. It has been most effective when awareness has been focused on the CNO as an interdisciplinary effort (Lamb, 1995, p. 22). Forums are used within the organization to give rapid feedback concerning the progress of the project and to share what is being learned. The public relations department has been invaluable (Lamb, 1995, p. 23). A CNO must handle enrollees with a variety of risks to survive financially; 80% should be those expected to stay healthy with few needs for acute or chronic services, and 20% should be moderate or high risk. Health promotion services must be provided to keep members active and functioning in the community; nutrition, exercise, and stress management are valued by the members. There must be a balance between providing services and saving money; each CNO provider (nurse partner) is responsible for designing the best service to achieve the individual's goals at the lowest cost with the help of a service delivery coordinator (Lamb, 1995, p. 23). Communication is the key to the CNO provider having the awareness needed to interpret redundant or conflicting information. Each part of the system must reinforce all others or the desired impact on quality and cost will not be realized (Lamb, 1995, p. 25). At Carondelet, they have found shifting to community-based care has required innovative thinking, professionals with different preparation, and increased collaboration and attention to how all the system parts work together (Lamb, 1995, p. 26).

CONCLUSION

This chapter provided examples from across the United States of community-based models of health care and agencies working together in the community. We have given examples and examined in detail a community heath center, home care programs, school-based clinics, and joint programs between the community and the hospital. Agencies do work together in the community, and the innovative community programs discussed included block nursing, parish nursing, and a nursing network. We ended with a brief description of the new Community Nursing Organization pilot program.

Chapter 10 will trace the history of medical education in the United States and examine medical care. Issues such as access to health care, physician responsibility, reimbursement, utilization management, and the future role of the physician are discussed.

REFERENCES

Abrams, R., Savela, T., Trinity, M. T., Falik, M., Tutunjian, B., and Ulmer, C. (1995). Performance of community health centers under managed care. *Journal of Ambulatory Medicine, 18*(3), 77–88.

Alford, R. R. (1975). *Health care politics.* Chicago: The University of Chicago Press.

Bellin, S. S., & Geiger, H. J. (1976). The impact of a neighborhood health center. In R. L. Kane, J. M. Kasteler, & R. M. Gray (Eds.), *The health gap* (pp. 178–201). New York: Springer.

Capitman, J. A., Haskins, B., & Bernstein, J. (1986). Case management approaches in coordinated community-oriented long-term care demonstrations. *The Gerontologist, 26*, 398–404.

Davis, I. L. (1992). Client identification and outreach: Case management in school-based services for teenage parents. In B. S. Vourlekis & R. R. Greene (Eds.), *Social casework management* (pp. 27–34). New York: Aldine De Gruyter.

Djupe, A. M. (1996). Parish nursing. In E. L. Cohen (Ed.), *Nurse case management in the 21st. Century* (pp. 140–148). St. Louis, MO: Mosby.

Drummond, M., Buss, T. F., & Ladigo, M. A. (1992). Volunteers for community health: An Ohio hospital sponsors parish nursing programs for area churches and synagogues. *Health Progress, 73*(5), 20–24.

Dunkle, R. M. (1996). Parish nurses help patients: Body and soul. *RN, 59*(5), 55–57.

Ethridge, P. (1991). A nursing HMO: Carondelet St. Mary's experience. *Nursing Management, 22*(7), 22–27.

Ethridge, P., & Lamb, G. S. (1989). Professional nursing case management improves quality, access and costs. *Nursing Management, 20*(3), 30–35.

Eustis, N., Greenberg, J., & Patten, S. (1984). *Long-term care for older persons: A policy perspective.* Monterey, CA: Brooks and Cole.

Grebin, B. (1994). Exclusive interview with Burton Grebin, MD. *The Remington Report, Aug/Sept,* 5–6.

Hare, I., & Clark, J. P. (1992). Case management assessment in school social work and early intervention programs for disabled infants and toddlers. In B. S. Vourlekis & R. R. Greene (Eds.), *Social casework management* (pp. 51–74). New York: Aldine De Gruyter.

Hawkins, J. E., & Higgins, L. P. (1993). *Nursing and the American health care delivery system* (4th ed.). New York: Tiresias.

Jamieson, M. K. (1987). Notes from the field: The St. Anthony Park block nurse program. *American Journal of Public Health, 77*(9), 1227–1228.

Jamieson, M. K. (1990). Block nursing: Practicing autonomous professional nursing in the community. *Nursing and Health Care, 1*, 250–253.

Jamieson, M. K. (1996). Grass roots efforts: Nurses involved in the political process. In E. L. Cohen (Ed.), *Nurse case management in the 21st. Century* (pp. 21–27). St. Louis, MO: Mosby.

Jamieson, M. K., & Martinson, I. (1983). Block nursing: neighbors caring for neighbors. *Nursing Outlook, 31*, 270–273.

Jenkins, M., & Torrisi, D. L. (1995). Nurse practitioners, community nursing center, and contracting for managed care. *Journal of the American Academy of Nurse Practitioners, 7*(3), 119–124.

Jerrell, J. M., & Hu, T. (1989). Cost-effectiveness of intensive clinical and case management compared with an existing system of care. *Inquiry, 26*(3), 224–234.

Jonas, J. M., & Banta, H. D. (1986). Government in the health care delivery system. In S. Jonas (Ed.), *Health care delivery system in the United States* (3rd ed., pp. 333–366). New York: Springer.

Jonas, S., & Rosenberg, S. N. (1986). Ambulatory care. In S. Jonas (Ed.), *Health care delivery system in the United States* (3rd ed., pp. 125–165). New York: Springer.

Kaplan, M. (1992). Care planning for children with HIV/AIDS: A family perspective. In B. S. Vourlekis & R. R. Greene (Eds.), *Social casework management* (pp. 75–88). New York: Aldine De Gruyter.

Kelly, K., & Maas, M. (1994). *Health care rationing: Dilemma and paradox.* St. Louis, MO: Mosby.

King, J. M., Lakin, J. A., & Striepe, J. (1993). Coalition building between public health nurses and parish nurses. *Journal of Nursing Administration, 23*(2), 27–31.

Klaw, S. (1975). *The great American medicine show.* New York: Penguin.

Lamb, G. S. (1995). Early lessons from a capitated community-based nursing model. *Nursing Administration Quarterly, 19*(3), 18–26.

Lamb, G. S., & Stempel, J. E. (1994). Nurse case management from the client's view: Growing as insider-expert. *Nursing Outlook, 42*(1), 7–13.

Lebow, G., & Kane, B. (1992). Assessment: Private case management with the elderly. In B. S. Vourlekis & R. R. Greene (Eds.), *Social work case management* (pp. 35–50). New York: Aldine De Gruyter.

Lumsdon, K. (1994, October 5). No place like home. *Hospitals & Health Networks*, pp. 45–52.

MacAdam, M., Capitman, J., Yee, D., Prottas, J., Leutz, W., & Westwater, D. (1989). Case management for frail elders: The Robert Wood Johnson Foundation's program for hospital initiative in long-term care. *Gerontologist, 29*, 737–744.

Martin, L. (1996). Parish nursing: Keeping body and soul together. *Canadian Nurse, 92*(1), 25–28.

Martinson, I. M., Jamieson, J. K., O'Grady, B., & Sime, M. (1985). The block nurse program. *Journal of Community Health Nursing, 2*(1), 21–29.

Meeker, R. J., DeAngelis, C., Berman, B., Freeman, H. E., & Oda, D. (1986). A comprehensive school health initiative. *Image: Journal for Nursing Scholarship, 18*(3), 86–91.

Michaels, C. (1992). Carondelet St. Mary's nursing enterprise. *Nursing Clinics of North America, 27*(1), 77–85.

Miller, M. A. (1995). Culture, spirituality, and women's health. *Journal of Obstetric, Gynecologic, and Neonatal Nursing, 24,* 257–263.

Miskelly, S. (1995). A parish nursing model: Applying the community health nursing process in a community church. *Journal of Community Health Nursing, 12*(1), 1–14.

Mor, V., Piette, J., & Fleishman, J. (1989). Community-based case management. *Health Affairs, 8,* 139–154.

Newman, M., Lamb, G., & Michaels, C. (1991). Nurse case management: The coming together of theory and practice. *Nursing and Health Care, 12,* 404–408.

Olson, D., Rickles, J., & Travlik, K. (1995). A treatment-team of managed mental health care. *Psychiatric Services, 46,* 252–256.

Operational Standards for Early Intervention Programs in Massachusetts. (1996). *Early intervention policy manual.* Boston: MDPH Bureau of Family and Community Health Division for Children with Special Needs EI Services.

Sardell, A. (1988). *The U.S. experiment in social medicine: The community health center program, 1965–1986.* Pittsburgh, PA: University of Pittsburgh Press.

Schank, M. J., Weis, D., & Matheus, R. (1996). Parish nursing: Ministry of healing. *Geriatric Nursing, 17*(1), 11–13.

Schorr, D. (1970). *Don't get sick in America.* Nashville, TN: Aurora.

Simington, J., Olson, J., & Douglas, L. (1996). Promoting well-being with a parish. *Canadian Nurse, 92*(1), 20–24.

Standard Service Contract for the Community Moms Project. (1995). *Service manual.* Boston: Department of Public Health.

CHAPTER 10

Physicians Learn New Roles for Managed Care: Modernizing the Caduceus

Carole Wieland Pearce and Carol J. McMahon Morin

Today, for the first time in many years, the physician is no longer unilaterally in charge of medical care. Third-party payers and managed care have wrestled away control, and physicians' roles have changed dramatically. Physicians, like everyone else in the health care system, are unsure of where they are going and what their roles will be.

In this chapter the evolution of medical education and medical care will be discussed, including the issues of access to care, personal responsibility of the physician, continuity of care, physician reimbursement, and utilization management. We will conclude with remarks regarding the future role of the physician.

MEDICAL EDUCATION

The history of medical education goes back to our earliest history as a nation. In Colonial days, many lay people were involved in medical care. In New England, the clergy, who were the best educated and most respected citizens, provided medical advice (Kaufman, 1976, p. 5). The physician was virtually a jack of all trades, providing services that ranged from surgery and mixing drugs to shaving beards, all without professional or legal constraints (Rogers, 1978, p. 15). Physicians were poorly educated and learned their profession through a 5-to 7-year apprenticeship (Kaufman, 1976, pp. 6–7). The United States did not wish to import the rigid caste system from Europe, which included well-established and professionally controlled medicine (Rogers, 1978, p. 15). The physicians who emigrated from Europe at that time tended to be either misfits or unsuccessful there (Kaufman, 1976, pp. 3, 5).

During the later Colonial period, a number of well-trained physicians arrived from Europe. These university-educated physicians proved to be excellent preceptors, and students soon desired more than rudimentary medical education. A small number of students even traveled to Europe to complete their education (Kaufman, 1976, pp. 8–10).

Gradually medicine changed. The first law regulating medicine was passed in New York in 1760; however, the law was only applicable in New York. Formal education consisted of anatomy lectures and demonstrations. Next, medical colleges were established as a step toward reform of medical education (Kaufman, 1976, pp. 13–14); the College of Philadelphia graduated the first medical class in 1768 (Kaufman, 1976, p. 21).

In the middle of the 19th century, physicians were educated in privately owned for-profit proprietary medical schools; only some universities trained doctors. The entrance requirements were the ability to pay and to read and write. Large numbers of physicians were trained; there were more physicians per capita then than now, and every small town had a physician. There were no standards for medical practice. As specialists arrived from Europe, they were critical of American proprietary medical education (Rogers, 1978, pp. 16–17). Reform of medical schools began slowly. The reforms included setting standards concerning length and content of medical education and the need for examinations (Kaufman, 1976, p. 87).

The actual improvement in the quality of medical education occurred after a study of medical school education carried out by the Carnegie Foundation for the Advancement of Teaching and the American Medical Association. The study findings were reported in 1910 in *The Flexner Report* (Johnson, 1978, p. xvii). Abraham Flexner, a schoolmaster from Louisville, Kentucky, visited 155 medical schools in the United States and Canada (Hudson, 1986, p. 1) and reported that medical education was a sham and recommended all proprietary medical schools close (Rogers, 1978, p. 16). Flexner (1910) recommended reducing the number and improving the quality of medical schools; those schools remaining should be within a university and located within a large city. States or regions should have medical schools based on need, and the overall number of medical school graduates should be diminished. Another recommendation was for development of expertise at specific locations, such as tropical medicine in New Orleans, Louisiana and occupational diseases in Pittsburgh, Pennsylvania. The report theorized that as more competent physicians were educated, the public health and physical status of wage earners would improve (pp. 143–155).

Dramatic changes in medical education followed. Ehrenreich and English (1973) stated:

> As for the smaller, poorer schools, which included most of the sectarian schools and special schools for blacks and women—Flexner did not consider them worth saving. Their options were to close, or to remain open and face public denunciation in the report Flexner was preparing. . . . In its wake (*Flexner Report*), medical schools closed by the score, including six of the American eight black medical schools and a majority of the 'irregular' (nontraditional) schools, which had been a haven for female students. (p. 30)

The proprietary schools closed (Rogers, 1978, pp. 16–17); many were in rural areas and the South (Ehrenreich & English, 1973, p. 30). Curricula were improved and licensing laws were established (Rogers, 1978, pp. 16–17).

At that time, the majority of the physicians were general practitioners, supplemented with a small group of specialists. Beginning in 1922, with the discovery of penicillin and the subsequent development of potent pharmacologics, increasing use of anesthesia, improved surgical techniques, and eventual development of synthetic replacements for the human body, the general practitioner could no longer deal with all aspects of patient care. The general public, now largely middle class, demanded consultations. Specialists, who were awarded higher status and more money, largely replaced the general practitioners (Rogers, 1978, pp. 16–17).

After 1960, changes again occurred in medicine. Thirty new medical schools opened, responding to the opportunity for reform and innovation. These schools are community-based medical schools and graduate mostly family or primary care physicians. Many of these medical schools do not have a university hospital and have found it necessary in keeping with the changing needs of clients to use community hospitals (Hunt, 1977, pp. 4–8).

Block, Clark-Chiarelli, Peters, and Singer (1996) found that despite this emphasis, medical students today are not encouraged to pursue primary care careers and feel overwhelmingly discouraged from becoming primary physicians. The third-and fourth-year medical students believed that generalists were not the best physicians to handle serious illnesses and viewed their primary care training as inferior to specialty training (p. 677). Only one sixth of medical schools require students to spend time working in a health maintenance organization (HMO) (Veloski, Barzansky, Nash, Bastacky, & Stevens, 1996, p. 667). Block et al., accusing physicians of professional prejudice (p. 682), concluded that, "If medical educators seek to optimize enthusiasm and preparation for primary care careers, they must develop approaches to changing the attitudes, values, and composition of their faculties" (p. 677).

It has been estimated that 75% of American medical school graduates become specialists (Ginzberg & Ostow, 1994, p. 45), and approximately 30% of physicians provide primary care (Drake, Fitzgerald, & Jaffe, 1993, p. 35). United States statistics show an increase in actual numbers of general or family physicians in office-based direct patient care since 1980, but a decrease in percentage. In 1970, 58,800 physicians (26.89%) were in general or family practice. By 1980, the number had decreased to 47,800 and the percentage to 17.62. Since then, the number of family and general physicians has increased, while the percentage decreased and the total number of physicians has increased (1985, 53,900 or 16.38%; 1990, 57,600 or 16.0%; and 1993, 58,100 or 14.57%). The total numbers of nonfederal office-based physicians were 329,000, 359,900, and 398,800, respectively (U.S. Department of Commerce, Bureau of the Census, 1995, p. 121). As managed care expands, the shortage of general practitioners is predicted to get worse (Wartman, 1994, p. 2540). However, if 40% to 65% of Americans enroll in managed care networks by the year 2000, a more than 60% excess in specialists is predicted (Weiner, 1994, p. 222).

MEDICAL CARE

Our present medical system grew out of concern for public health and disease prevention in the 19th century. Diseases were primarily caused by adverse living conditions, poor sanitation, contaminated water supplies, imported products, and other similar concerns. Those issues dominated the concerns of medicine until the early 1900s. Medicine in the United States was not based on a sound, scientific base and was quite primitive; medical education was based on apprenticeships or training in poor quality institutions (Johnson, 1978, p. xvi).

By the early 19th century, much of medical care consisted of treatment that later came to be regarded as torture—bleeding, leeches, cupping, purging, and sweating. Treatment was based on depletion by bloodletting or stimulation by medication (Kaufman, 1976, p. 57). In New England, the Thomson method of cure consisted of steaming a patient by a fire or coals and administration of botanical drugs (herbs) (Kaufman, 1976, p. 65). Allopathy (active intervention to counteract disease and injury as practiced by most physicians in the United States today) (Glanze, Anderson, & Anderson, 1990, p. 44) and homeopathy (therapy that reinforced the body's own healing by use of very small doses of medicine) (Glanze et al., p. 574) thrived as did eclectic medicine (Kaufman, 1976, pp. 69–70).

Boards of health were first established in the mid-1800s, and in 1879 a largely powerless National Board of Health was formed. The country was responding to widespread epidemics of malaria, smallpox, tuberculosis, yellow fever, typhoid, typhus, and cholera (Johnson, 1978, p. xvi).

Medicine began to emerge as a scientific discipline and a political force by the beginning of the 20th century. The American Medical Association (AMA) became the voice for physicians, even though it had been in existence since 1847. The scientific foundation of medicine was reinforced by the new emphasis on experimental research; increasing specialization was promoted (Johnson, 1978, p. xvi). Most physicians were general practitioners, but many focused on a specialty part-time. This tendency toward specialization has continued (Johnson, 1978, p. xvii).

Today, once again medicine is changing with a mandate from the federal government to produce more physicians who are generalists and diminish the number of physicians who have specialty training. The large academic medical centers, which produced excellent specialists, cannot as easily produce generalists (Rogers, 1978, p. 43). Total medical care is increasingly delivered in the suburbs (Rogers, 1978, p. 70), and there is increasing emphasis on the social sciences as a necessary part of medical education (Fein, 1987, p. 65).

Physicians, who were in charge of medicine, are now in increasing numbers becoming employees whose practices are strongly influenced by third-party payers, HMOs, preferred provider organizations (PPOs), and state and federal governments' guidelines and restrictions.

ACCESS TO CARE

Physicians have traditionally controlled access to care, to treatment itself, decisions concerning treatment, hospitalization, and referral to other providers. They were self-employed and members of a medical staff at a hospital, which had its own bylaws, communication system, and organization. Physicians practiced solo or in a group and held admission privileges at a given hospital or more than one hospital. Because physicians were not hospital employees, they were not under direct supervision of the hospital administrators. The medical staff was able to sanction, influence, or modify a physician's practice. Insurance companies could either pay for the care or challenge the physician's decisions concerning the need for care (Merwin, 1994, p. 65). This resulted in a very expensive health care delivery system. Managed care is slowing the inflation of health care costs and is changing the manner in which health care is delivered, and the physician is directly affected.

Access to health care should not be limited by the gatekeeping of managed care, but should be facilitated by expert selection of appropriate services (Rosenthal, Riemenschneider, & Feather, 1996, p. 341). Geographically, we have unequal access to care. There are ample physicians in this country (250 physicians per 100,000 population) (Ginzberg & Ostow, 1994, p. 45). However, the ratio of physicians to rural areas is askew. Metropolitan areas in this country have four to five times more physicians than rural areas. This overabundance of physicians in urban areas may be attributed to the unwillingness of physicians to practice in rural areas (McPhee, 1984, p. 19).

PERSONAL RESPONSIBILITY OF THE PHYSICIAN

"The essential spirit of the physician–patient relationship is in potential jeopardy in managed care" (Perkel, 1996, 272). The physician's ultimate moral and legal responsibility for those entrusted for care has not changed, even though the insurance companies and managed care have put strict constraints on length of hospital stay, surgical treatment, diagnostic tests, and so on. With managed care, physicians are no longer able to merely handle their patients the way they wish. Limitations are placed on them. Physicians believe they are losing their autonomy and fear rationing of care; they believe these changes interfere with their individual decision-making ability and affect the quality of the care they are able to provide (Capuzzi, 1994, pp. 82–83). Vanderveer and Kelly (1996) found that physicians working in managed care worked longer hours and faced more demands from their patients (p. 822).

As an example, in California physicians were held responsible for the amputation of a woman's leg. They failed to file a request for additional hospitalization days after a 4-day extension expired, and the woman was discharged. She did poorly at home, was admitted on an emergency basis, and attempts to save her leg were futile. The physicians should have requested an extension during the woman's initial hospitalization. The physician cannot merely blame the insurance company for limiting the hospital stay (Brent, 1991, pp. 8–9).

In spite of resisting managed care, many physicians have signed up with managed care plans, especially with PPOs (Taylor & Morrison, 1993, p. 66). The actual number is unavailable because the U.S. Department of

Commerce, Bureau of Statistics does not have a category for managed care. Those physicians who remain in private practice tend to join group practices (Rosenfield, 1994, p. 1).

CONTINUITY OF CARE

Continuity of care is important regardless of the delivery system. Physicians, like nurses, social workers, and physical therapists, can do their job best when relationships are developed with the patients over time. Physicians can identify subtle changes, and patients will provide more complete information to persons they trust. This relationship provides direct and indirect benefits over time to both patient and physician (Falk & Bower, 1994, p. 168). Physicians, payors, and patients must form a partnership for care to occur on a continuum (Falk & Bower, 1994, p. 169). A collaborative team, with the physician as team member, is the best way for patients to have continuity of care.

PAYMENT TO THE PHYSICIAN

The payment methods for the physician vary greatly, as do the details within the types of payment. The traditional fee-for-service method of physician payment is becoming obsolete; with managed care, a variety of methods of payment are utilized. Dr. J. Heyman in a *Boston Globe* article is quoted as saying, "With fee-for-service, physicians are paid for what they do. Under some managed care plans, they are paid for what they don't do" (Pham, 1996, p. E1).

In fee-for-service arrangements, the physician establishes a charge for a procedure or service and then collects payment from the insurance company, government, or person who receives the service. The incentive is for the physician to cut costs for the procedure or service, but there is no incentive to minimize the number of services or procedures. Actually, the more services provided, the more personal revenue is generated (Held & Reinhardt, 1980, p. 5). Traditionally specialists' incomes have been larger than general practitioners. It has been estimated that specialists earn approximately twice that of generalists (Ginzberg, 1994, p. 46). Physician incomes have skyrocketed with the fee-for-service payment method (Taylor & Morrison, 1993, p. 66). The golden age of doctors' incomes was in the 1980s; this included the early managed care systems that were then still largely fee-for-service arrangements (Taylor & Morrison, 1993, p. 66).

Today, managed care provides a variety of mechanisms for payment to physicians. PPOs use discounted charges, relative value systems, negotiated fee schedules, and capitation (Schmitt, 1989, pp. 52–56); HMOs pay salaries and utilize provider risk pools. In HMOs, there are incentives for efficiency and smallest total cost per enrollee (Hicks, Stallmeyer, & Coleman, 1993, pp. 28–29). As managed care developed alternative mechanisms for payment to physicians, many have taken serious cuts in income. On the other hand, they have gained in personal, family, and educational time.

The variety of managed care plans and accompanying payment plans appears unlimited. The following is a summary of some of the methods of physician payment under managed care today; undoubtedly tomorrow will bring more creative ways to cut health care costs.

1.   Capitation pays the physician a fixed amount per member per month and provides services; the incentive is to minimize costs, thereby pocketing the balance (Hicks et al., 1993, p. 26). This method may undermine trust in physicians (Selker, 1996, p. 450).

2.   Discounted charges means a lower fee is paid for each service; there is the same basic incentive structure as fee for services (Hicks et al., 1993, p. 27).

3.   Relative value system fees are paid based on the relative worth of one procedure or service multiplied by a conversion factor or price multipliers set by the payer (Schmitt, 1989, p. 53); this payment method can lead to inefficient and skewed services (Hicks et al., 1993, p. 27).

4.   Negotiated fee is a specific fee paid for a specific service (Schmitt, 1989, p. 54) where overall utilization is not limited; certain services at certain sites are encouraged, that is, a procedure performed on an outpatient basis pays more than the same procedure performed on an inpatient basis (Hicks et al., 1993, p. 27).

5.   Salary structure means the physician is an employee and is paid a specific amount by contract; there is no incentive to alter practice, but bonuses may be awarded for productivity (Hicks et al., 1993, p. 28; Pham, 1996).

6.   Risk pool holds back a percentage (5% to 50%) of salary or fee-for-service receipts and distributes the money (perhaps at the end of the year based on performance). This method uses peer pressure and rewards individual or group efficiency (Hicks et al., 1993, p. 28; Pham, 1996).

Patients have a right to know the details of these arrangements.

UTILIZATION MANAGEMENT

Care provided by specialists is typically more expensive than care provided by generalists; specialists have been shown to rely more heavily on costly tests, medications, and hospitalizations than do family and general practitioners (Drake et al., 1993, p. 35). Because physicians have been responsible for more than 88% of health care costs, either directly or indirectly, changing their behavior is critical to the success of managed care (Kent & Roberts, 1989, p. 101). Quality of care must be considered along with cost savings. Physicians must be actively involved in decision making and supported by clinical authority figures (Milstein, Bergthold, & Selbovitz, 1993, p. 373). Physicians are accountable to the managed care plan in a way they never were under fee-for-service plans.

Physicians' ways of practicing are directly affected by utilization control. In addition to financial incentives, managed care plans include some type of mandated utilization control. Utilization management is "the ability of providers and insurers to control cost and enhance the quality of and access to care for patients through efficient management and provision of medical services" (Kent & Roberts, 1989, p. 103) or " . . . deliberate action to induce a more economical mix of treatment without sacrificing health outcomes" (Milstein et al., 1993, p. 372). Effective utilization management plans are: (a) prospective, requiring preadmission certification, preauthorization, second opinion; (b) concurrent review, involving admission review, length of stay review, monitoring of individual patient's treatment plan, discharge planning; and (c) retrospective review, a review of treatment after services are provided (Hicks et al., 1993, pp. 30–32).

Effective utilization management can be accomplished by careful selection of physicians, educating physicians in the treatment techniques that are most cost effective, and providing financial incentives, penalties, or both to alter physician behavior. Utilization review should be carried out by an independent professional (Milstein et al., 1993, pp. 372–376).

Efficient utilization can be accomplished by selection of appropriate physicians with efficient utilization in their practices and inducing preferential use of them. As much as 10% can be saved by eliminating inefficient physicians. If initially a physician is given provisional membership, it is not as difficult to terminate for inefficiency as it would be for a full member. The present methods for judging physician utilization are to use claims, medical records, and hospital discharge data (Milstein et al., 1993, pp. 372–373). Obtaining this information without the use of computerized records is expensive and time consuming, however.

Education of the physician is the second method of utilization management. There is evidence that feedback concerning the individual or group utilization and cost is ineffective in inducing efficiency unless it is accompanied by incentives. Feedback of utilization data accompanied by potential incentives or sanctions is useful if the physician finds the data and analyses credible (O'Grady, 1993, p. 396). If necessary, concrete evidence of excessive orders must be presented (Milstein et al., 1993, pp. 373–374). Individual performance data provide physicians with information that allows them to compare their performances with their peers and with the norms and standards of their profession or managed care. When physicians fail to modify their behavior, discipline and sanctions may be necessary to effect change (Hicks et al., 1993, p. 33).

Use of incentive or penalties is the third way managed care controls cost. Audits for financial recovery detect overuse and fraud (O'Grady, 1993, p. 397). In a study of a managed care ambulatory setting, physicians were asked to refund overpayment when misuse of procedure codes or errors were detected in billing. Those who refused were asked to resign. The per member cost was 16% less than for nonmembers (Roberts & Zalta, 1993, p. 391). Perhaps the most useful levers for utilization are financial incentives and disincentives, although physicians tend to be risk aversive and mistrustful of data and management. Shifting more of the financial risk to the physician is effective. Health plans cannot afford physicians who overuse resources (Petersen, 1993, p. 78). Deselection is not considered the appropriate lever to use in utilization issues, but may be needed at times and provides evidence to physicians that it will be used if needed (O'Grady, 1993, pp. 396–397). Discipline is a punitive way to change their behavior; education is a better method (Hicks et al., 1993, p. 33).

MEDICAID

Many physicians have been reluctant to care for persons with Medicaid coverage due to low reimbursement rates and high overhead costs (Witek & Hostage, 1994, p. 62); payments may also be delayed. To cut costs, Medicaid began limiting physicians' services by type of procedure or number of visits (Davis, Anderson, Rowland, & Steinberg, 1990, p. 80). Medicaid continues to strain state and federal budgets; the response has been managed care Medicaid programs. Almost every state either has such a program or has one in development (Witek & Hostage, 1994, p. 62). However, Medicaid managed care has found it difficult to attract providers due to the high risk nature of this population (Witek & Hostage, 1994, pp. 63–64).

THE FUTURE: THE ROLE OF THE PHYSICIAN IN THE COMMUNITY

"The physician in the past was ignorant, empirical, wonderfully generous and beloved (mostly) by his patients; the physician of the present is less ignorant, less empirical, and all too often considerably less generous and not at all beloved. But what about the physician of tomorrow?" (Chapman, 1987, p. 55). No one could have foreseen what has happened today in medicine and to the physician personally. No one can predict the future with any degree of certainty, but surely elements discussed here will in some way be part of the future.

Physicians are worried about their place in society and their part of the economic pie. Physicians believe there are already too many doctors and that they will all be harmed unless physician manpower is controlled (Moore, 1995, p. 14; Sullivan, Watanabe, Whitcomb, & Kindig, 1996, p. 704). There is concern regarding increasing numbers of international medical school graduates in residency training programs (Salsberg, Wing, Dionne, & Jemiolo, 1996, pp. 683, 688). Physician salaries dropped for the first time in more than 10 years in 1994, although they are still among the highest paid workers. Specialist salaries have dropped the most (Meckler, 1996, pp. 2, 8). Another concern is the diversion of health care dollars by HMOs. Physicians also wish to control nurse practitioners and are lobbying to prevent enactment of laws allowing them to provide medical care without a physician's direct supervision (Moore, 1995, p. 14).

The physician's office, often located in the community, is now a major port of entry to the health care system. Emergency rooms, clinics, and others also provide entry. The physician's office is likely to remain a major port of entry. Physicians will need to be reimbursed for time spent managing patients in the community. The physician will hire a nurse or social worker as case manager to handle the holistic needs of the clients who need such services; the case manager may be the employee of the physician or a vendor who provides service on a contractual basis. Capitation will enable the physicians to make those choices specific to the needs of their practices.

The trend toward physicians as employees will continue. They will continue to be employed in walk-in centers, community health centers, emergency rooms, hospitals, and similar arrangements. The physician will work for an HMO or other managed care system. The physician will also be called in as a paid consultant in the nurse–social worker managed care centers in the community.

The physician will be a team member in the community and may not be the one in charge of the team. The person who leads the team should be the person most qualified to meet the holistic health needs of the client, family, or group. When community physicians no longer feel it necessary to be in control of all medical care, they will become better team players on a team in which each member has an equally important contribution to the total planning, implementation, and evaluation of care.

Informatics networks will enable the physicians to review the status of hospitalized patients, find innovative treatments, query insurance coverage, order the drugs, schedule a consultation, reserve operating rooms, and order follow-up lab work without ever leaving their offices. This entire scenario might take 1 hour as compared with several hours of both physician and staff time.

Telemedicine today enables physicians at large medical centers to examine and treat patients at satellite locations, aiding isolated communities in delivering optimum care at the local site (Sanders & Tedesco, 1994, p. 31). More widespread use of this technology can improve the quality of care in the community and allow patients to be cared for near home. Will this also increase the cost of medical care?

Medical education will continue its trend toward educating physicians to be educated persons and humane physicians.

In the concluding chapter, we will share our vision of how nursing and social work, through collaboration, can prepare to meet the challenge of managed care of tomorrow. Three areas require particular attention: education of social workers and nurses, examination of ethics and values for health professionals in a managed care environment, and formation of interdisciplinary research teams who will examine the processes and outcomes in a health care system that is increasingly dominated by managed care.

REFERENCES

Block, S. D., Clark-Chiarelli, N., Peters, A. S., & Singer, J. D. (1996). Academia's chilly climate for primary care. *Journal of the American Medical Association, 276*, 677–682.

Brent, N. J. (1991). Managed care: Legal and ethical implications. *Home Healthcare Nurse, 9*(1), 8–10.

Brocato, F. M., Trapp, R. G., & Scalia, C. L. (1993). Florida Gulf Coast Health Coalition: Employer analysis pro forma. In P. Boland (Ed.), *Making managed healthcare work: A practical guide to strategies and solutions* (pp. 369–370). New York: McGraw-Hill.

Capuzzi, C. (1994). Consumer, provider, and third-party payor perspectives of health care rationing. In K. Kelly & M. Mass (Eds.), *Health care rationing: Dilemma and paradox* (pp. 75–94). St. Louis: Mosby.

Chapman, C. B. (1987). Medical education: The physician—then, now, and tomorrow. In C. Vevier (Ed.), *Flexner: 75 years later* (pp. 47–62). Lanham, MD: University Press of America.

Davis, K., Anderson, G. F., Rowland, D., & Steinberg, E. P. (1990). *Health care cost containment*. Baltimore: Johns Hopkins University Press.

Drake, D., Fitzgerald, S., & Jaffe, M. (1993). *Hard choices: Healthcare at what cost?* Kansas City, MO: Andrews & McMeel.

Ehrenreich, B., & English, D. (1973). *Witches, midwives and nurse: A history of women healers*. Old Westbury, NY: Feminist Press.

Falk, C. D., & Bower, K. A. (1994). Managing care across department, organization, and setting boundaries. In K. Kelly & M. Mass (Eds.), *Health care rationing: Dilemma and paradox* (pp. 161–176). St. Louis, MO: Mosby.

Fein, R. (1987). Medical education: The impact of the social sciences on a changing delivery system. In C. Vevier (Ed.), *Flexner: 75 years later* (pp. 63–75). Lanham, MD: University Press of America.

Flexner, A. (1910). *Medical education in the United States and Canada: A report to the Carnegie Foundation for the Advancement of Teaching*. Washington, DC: Science and Health Publications, Inc.

Ginzberg, E., & Ostow, M. (1994). *The road to reform: the future of health care in America*. New York: Free Press.

Glanze, W. D., Anderson, K. N., & Anderson, L. E. (Eds.). (1990). *Mosby's medical, nursing, and allied health dictionary* (3rd ed.). St. Louis, MO: Mosby.

Held, P. J., & Reinhardt, U. E. (1980). Prepaid medical practice: A summary of findings from a recent survey of group practices in the United States. *Group Health Journal, 1*(2), 4–15.

Hicks, L. L., Stallmeyer, J. M., & Coleman, J. R. (1993). *Role of the nurse in managed care*. Washington, DC: American Nurses Publishing.

Hudson, R. P. (1986). Abraham Flexner in historical perspective. In B. Barzansky & N. Gevitz (Eds.), *Beyond Flexner: Medical eduction in the twentieth century*. New York: Greenwood.

Hunt, A. D. (1977). A time of change and reform in medical education. In A. D. Hunt & L. E. Weeks (Eds.), *Medical education since 1960: Marching to a different drummer* (pp. 2–9). E. Lansing, MI: Michigan State University Foundation and the W. K. Kellogg Foundation.

Johnson, S. C. (1978). Introduction: Perspectives on the Health Policy process. In R. M. Battistella & T. G. Rundall (Eds.), *Health care policy in a changing environment* (pp. xv–xxvii). Berkeley, CA: McCutchan Publishing.

Kaufman, M. (1976). *American medical education: The formative years, 1765–1910*. Westport, CT: Greenwood Press.

Kent, M. S. & Roberts, N. (1989). Utilization management. In D. L. Cobbs (Ed.), *Preferred provider organizations: Strategies for sponsors and network providers*. Chicago: American Hospital Publishing, Inc.

McPhee, J. (1984). *Heirs of general practice*. New York: Noonday Press.

Meckler, L. (1996). Doctors experience rare salary reduction. *Duke University Chronicle, September 4,* 2, 8.

Merwin, E. I. (1994). Accountability for allocation of health care resources: Is the fox guarding the henhouse? In K. Kelly & M. Mass (Eds.), *Health care rationing: Dilemma and paradox* (pp. 55–71). St. Louis, MO: Mosby.

Milstein, A., Bergthold, L., & Selbovitz, L. (1993). Utilization review techniques. In P. Boland (Ed.), *Making managed healthcare work: A practical guide to strategies and solutions* (pp. 371–388). New York: McGraw-Hill.

Moore, J. D. (1995). AMA members target managed care. *Modern Healthcare, June,* 14.

O'Grady, K. F. (1993). Physician utilization profiling: The key to managing ambulatory utilization. In P. Boland (Ed.), *Making managed healthcare work: A practical guide to strategies and solutions* (pp. 394–399). New York: McGraw-Hill.

Perkel, R. L. (1996). Ethics and managed care. *Medical Clinics of North America, 80,* 263–278.

Petersen, W. E. (1993). Provider perspective. In P. Boland (Ed.), *Making managed healthcare work: A practical guide to strategies and solutions* (pp. 78–79). New York: McGraw-Hill.

Pham, A. (1996). Fee systems may affect doctor care. *The Boston Globe.* August 11, pp. E1, E15.

Roberts, N., & Zalta, E. (1993). CAPP CARE: Utilization review of ambulatory services. In P. Boland (Ed.), *Making managed healthcare work: A practical guide to strategies and solutions* (pp. 389–391). New York: McGraw-Hill.

Rogers, D. E. (1978). *American medicine: Challenges for the 1980s.* Cambridge, MA: Ballinger Publishing.

Rosenfield, R. H. (1994). Replacing the workshop model. *Topics in Health Care Financing, 20*(4), 1–15.

Rosenthal, T. C., Riemenschneider, T. A., & Feather, J. (1996). Preserving the patient referral process in the managed care environment. *American Journal of Medicine, 100,* 338–343.

Salsberg, E. S., Wing, P., Dionne, M. G., & Jemiolo, D. J. (1996). Graduate medical education and physician supply in New York State. *Journal of the American Medical Association, 276,* 683–688.

Sanders, J. H., & Tedesco, F. J. (1994, August/September). Telemedicine: Bringing medical care to isolated communities. *Remington Report,* pp. 31–34.

Schmitt, J. P. (1989). Provider payment systems. In D. L. Cobbs (Ed.), *Preferred provider organizations: Strategies for sponsors and network providers.* Chicago: American Hospital Publishing.

Selker, H. P. (1996). Capitated payment for medical care and the role of the physician. *Annals of Internal Medicine, 124*(4), 449–451.

Sullivan, R. B., Watanabe, M., Whitcomb, M. E., & Kindig, D. A. (1996). The evolution of divergences in physician supply policy in Canada and the United States. *Journal of the American Medical Association, 276,* 704–709.

Taylor, H., & Morrison, J. I. (1993). Attitudes toward managed healthcare. In P. Boland (Ed.), *Making managed healthcare work: A practical guide to strategies and solutions* (pp. 51–69). New York: McGraw-Hill.

U.S. Department of Commerce, Bureau of the Census. (1995). *Statistical Abstracts of the United States* (115th ed., p. 121). Washington, DC: U.S. Government Printing Office.

Vanderveer, R. B., & Kelly, D. J. (1996). U.S. Physicians respond to managed care. *Spectrum Health Care Delivery and Economics, August 6*, 821–829.

Veloski, J., Barzansky, B., Nash, D. B., Bastacky, S., & Stevens, D. P. (1996). Medical students education in managed care settings: Beyond health maintenance organizations (HMOs). *Journal of the American Medical Association, 276*, 667–671.

Wartman, S. A. (1994). Managed care and its effect on residency training in internal medicine. *Archives of Internal Medicine, 154*, 2539–2544.

Weiner, J. P. (1994). Forecasting the effects of health reform on US physician workforce requirement: Evidence from HMO staffing patterns. *Journal of the American Medical Association, 272*, 222–230.

Witek, J. E., & Hostage, J. L. (1994). Medicaid managed care: Problems and promise. *Journal of Ambulatory Medicine, 17*(1), 61–69.

CHAPTER 11

Getting It Together: Concluding Thoughts, Common Voices

In this book we have traced the historic antecedents and evolution of collaboration between social work and nursing and the impact of managed care on the potential for collaboration in the 21st century. Through our interviews, we have elicited the realities and dreams of collaboration, and the themes shared by our participants have led to the development of the Biopsychosocial Individual and Systems Intervention Model (BISIM). We have then operationalized the model through actual cases of collaboration in the community.

In view of the established need for collaboration, there are three areas that require attention by both social work and nursing: education; ethics and values for health care professionals in a managed care environment; and interdisciplinary research to underlie and advance practice and examine outcomes of care in an increasingly complex and technologically sophisticated system.

EDUCATION

Because the underlying thesis of the BISIM is collaboration, nurses and social workers most logically should be educated together. If collaboration is part of the educational foundation for practice for both professions, it follows that we should socialize students in their theoretical and clinical preparation to recognize and use their complementary skills and knowledge. As health care returns to the community, opportunities for educating these professionals together are easier to create.

Both professions need preparation for practicing in interdisciplinary teams. Both need to inculcate advocacy skills as an integral part of their professional psyches. Practice as case managers, as well as learning the theoretical underpinnings for the role, is essential preparation for both professionals for practice today. Creating measurable goals and strategies for measuring outcomes is essential to our survival as professions.

Both nursing and social work need to prepare their graduates with skills in informatics; independent functioning and accountability; and interdisciplinary collaboration and consultation with a community-aggregate focus. Nurses are accustomed to practicing with protocols; this is driven, in part, by state nurse practice acts. Social workers are beginning to develop protocols as they struggle to define and operationalize what they do so they can then spell out goals and measure outcomes of their practice. As we develop collaborative models for practice, we can create protocols together to guide our practice. Similarly, because it is difficult to determine who is responsible for what in patient outcomes, we certainly need to work together to identify goals with our clients and then design outcomes measures.

Education at the entry level is one responsibility of a profession. Equally important is reeducation of seasoned professionals who need skills and knowledge in new areas such as informatics, case management, and practice across settings or in new settings such as the community. More than two thirds of nurses have worked in hospitals over the past few decades. Many of these nurses will be displaced as hospitals merge and downsize. Similarly, social workers have often chosen institutional practice and are being displaced by shorter lengths of stay, downsizing of institutions, the fiscally driven push to return clients to the community as quickly as possible, and the press for ever shorter interventions in community settings.

In these two practice disciplines, single investigator research is becoming displaced by intradisciplinary and interdisciplinary models. The complex nature of systems, diseases, and human response patterns demands both a broad brush and many pigments for designing studies to answer questions of primary importance to changing and guiding practice. In educating social workers and nurses for a variety of levels of participation in research, we might consider collaborative models between the two professions. Perhaps then in the real world of practice, the seeds for collaborative research will take root. Certainly there are many examples of research by the two professions from their early days to the present.

Whether education is of those studying to become social workers or nurses or the reeducation of the seasoned professionals, similar areas need to be addressed for nurses and social workers to survive, thrive, and take charge of the future of both nursing and social work as the community more and more becomes the focus for their work. Many colleges and universities still do not educate their students adequately in the areas of advocacy, interdisciplinary collaboration, consultation, independent functioning, aggregate-community focus, protocol development, case management, informatics, quality assurance, health promotion and primary care, health policy and reform, and politics. It is time for education to be more innovative in the educational training settings; homeless residences, battered women's programs, school systems, prisons, the welfare system, and others are all possibilities (Donner, 1996, pp. 326–330).

ADVOCACY

Throughout our history, social workers and nurses have been advocates for patients. The advocate creates a climate for the individual, family, or group to act in its own best interest. If they are unable, the nurse or social worker takes on the cause. The advocate is ideally the case manager who acts on behalf of the client, defends the cause of the client, and supports the client in meeting goals. The advocate identifies cases, fosters independence, educates in use of resources and services, and encourages appropriate decision making. Consideration and respect for generational and cultural factors are crucial in this role (Davis, 1996, pp. 192–193).

COLLABORATION

Nurses and social workers in collaboration can plan and deliver high quality care to clients in the community. This will be accomplished by interdisciplinary teams of professionals working together. Learning to work together will benefit the members of the community, but also may help assure their survival as professionals. Holistic health care is integration of health care and is only possible with collaboration of the caregivers.

The purpose of collaboration in the community is "to build relationships with both care providers and patients, orchestrate their interaction and facilitate service utilization, all in an effort to keep people healthy and accident free" (Salzman, 1996, p. 10). With integrated care, there are no barriers to receiving treatment because the most appropriate care is received from the most qualified provider. The key is continuous communication among providers (Ramay, 1996, p. 20).

Low-income persons are most at risk, and we must make sure they have access to and quality of care. Low-income persons have a disproportionate incidence of children with physical growth disability and mental disability and childhood accidental injury, death, and drug involvement. Violence and victimization are expensive for all of us (Poole, 1995, pp. 164–165). Long-term care will be increasingly shifted to family and friends (Poole, 1995, p. 163). Nurses and social workers must be taught to design programs to deliver comprehensive health care to special populations and those either ill served or underserved today (Poole, 1995, p. 164). We can expect improved outcomes with a direct focus on population-based management (Shamansky, 1995, pp. 211–212). Increasingly, nurses and social workers will be caring for those with complex chronic illnesses in the community, and they will take care of them throughout the continuum of care (Berkman, 1996, p. 543) and for their entire lives.

CONSULTATION

The nurse and the social worker are the health care experts in the community; they have been active in public health, at the workplace, in the schools, and at home. They increasingly serve as consultants to other professionals in developing the multidisciplinary teams who will coordinate and deliver high quality care (Malloy, 1995, pp. 81–82).

Social workers are often educated with a macro focus, often falling under the category of social work administration. They learn about social planning, program evaluation, fiscal management, change strategy, information systems, community theory, research, grant writing, public policy, and so forth (McNutt, 1995, pp. 62–63, 70–71). Nursing administration students also learn about these macro issues; however, all nurses and social workers need this education.

Those who are preparing to become social workers or nurses and those who are already professionals must be prepared to be the consultants as health care is increasingly delivered in the community by a variety of agencies and community centers. Their collective experience and knowledge place them in the forefront for delivery of individual, holistic, appropriate, and cost-effective care in community settings. Agencies will increasingly use trained workers for much of the actual care delivery; however, that care cannot be planned, delivered, and evaluated without consulting the social workers and nurses.

INDEPENDENT FUNCTIONING

Nurses and social workers have the opportunity to function independently in the community. Working together to establish independent neighborhood wellness centers will allow clients to maintain their highest level of functioning, preserve independence and dignity, and enhance self-care (Hey, 1993, pp. 26–27). These centers need not be restricted to elderly clients, but can be like the settlement houses of long ago that provided care for the entire family. At such centers, education, screening, immunization, monitoring (such as height and weight, blood pressure, blood sugars, and cholesterol) and evaluation of episodic conditions can take place. Referrals can be made to physicians as needed (Hey, 1993, pp. 27–28). Home health care is an important part of nurses and social workers caring for people where they live in the community.

Students in social work and nursing must receive their educational preparation with a strong emphasis on independent functioning and health care in the community. Many need to be reeducated to effectively administer care with a community focus. In southeastern Massachusetts, a consortium consisting of home health care agencies, acute care hospitals, and a college of nursing joined forces to ensure that nurses remained actively employed. A program was designed to meet the reeducation needs of acute care nurses who wished to make the transition to the community. A local college provided the necessary education through the continuing education department (Smith & Shiner, 1996, pp. 33, 34, 36). The same model could be used for social workers.

AGGREGATE-COMMUNITY FOCUS

Social workers and nurses must learn to approach health care with focus on a group or the community. What are the most pressing health problems within a given community? How can those health needs be met best? More nurses and social workers can learn to make community assessments, plan for improving overall health of the community, carry out the plans, and evaluate success or failure and determine the next step(s) for solving the problems.

Each community or neighborhood has unique needs; the community with considerable low-income housing has different needs from those communities with predominantly blue collar workers or those known for their affluence. Yet, each has health care issues that need resolving. Vulnerable at-risk populations (people infected with HIV; abused children and adults; victims of domestic violence; pediatric oncology, mentally ill, and elderly patients) within the community are of great concern (Berkman, 1996, p. 548). Case finding, education, support groups, referrals, and a multitude of other services must be readily available within the community. We must take into account the cultural, psychosocial, spiritual, and environmental dimensions of health care. Nurses and social workers together can be the flexible creative leaders needed to deal with the complexities of health care in the community today and tomorrow (Berkman, 1996, p. 549).

Education in health promotion and illness prevention are part of this picture. Promoting a healthy lifestyle can reduce chronic illness and disability and save money (Poole, 1995, p. 164). Prevention will lower the need for services. To successfully accomplish these goals, integration of the myriad of services must occur, and relationships must be built between clients and care givers. Learning ways to attain and maintain wellness is the responsibility of both the community and the individual (Salzman, 1996, pp. 11–13). Screening is needed to identify those at risk for physical, psychological, social, or environmental need (Berkman et al., 1996, p. 2).

PROTOCOL DEVELOPMENT

During graduate education in nursing, educators often assign students to write health care protocols based on an extensive literature search, existing protocols, and algorithms. Protocols are important and useful for professional nurses and social workers. Learning to write them, separately and together, should be an integral part of education and reeducation of social workers and nurses. Our planning must include clearly defined goals that will form the basis for determining the effectiveness of the interventions (Strom & Gingerich, 1993, p. 80). Protocols will help provide the holistic care patients and their families desire.

CASE MANAGEMENT

Case management provides the opportunity for the social worker or nurse to provide health care on a continuum, that is, to bridge the gap between hospital and home or other care facilities and services. Both nurses and social workers are ideally suited to this role and educating them for the case management role is the starting point. At minimum, education should include advocacy, assessment, planning, monitoring, brokering, linkage, and evaluation (Kurtz, Bagarozzi, & Pollane, 1984, pp. 202, 205). Students need to train in managed care and case management. Dual case management should be considered (social worker and nurse sharing case management).

Case management for elderly persons, particularly in the community, is important in prevention of hospitalization. They need to learn how to recognize changes that indicate a need to call the physician. Visiting in the home is one way to accomplish this, and the frequency of the visits is determined by the individual client's particular needs. The case manager may administer physical care, psychosocial care, or both (Hey, 1993, pp. 29–31). Case management will benefit pregnant women, new parents, parents with troubled or problem children, ill children, and many others as well.

INFORMATICS

Today all students and professionals must be able to use computers for data entry, retrieval, and management. For truly collaborative and integrated care, communication must be continuous and efficient. Computers with appropriate software can provide the link within the provider system. Health care providers should be able to determine insurance coverage, access diagnostic information, make appointments with another providers, and write clinical notes; a computerized data management system is a great time and money saver (Ramay, 1996, pp. 20–21). "Integrating care within a comprehensive, full-service network allows the practitioner to provide the care they deem appropriate within the parameters of utilization and quality review, while at the same time reducing administrative costs" (Ramay, 1996, p. 21).

With a portable computer and telephone access, the nurse or social worker in the field can access needed information and provide immediate updates for client records. Provisions to insure privacy of individual record information are crucial. Careful software evaluation should be carried out before a purchase is made to ensure the program is able to meet the needs of the agency and the care givers.

QUALITY ASSURANCE

Along with managed care has come concern regarding the quality of health care. Consumer dissatisfaction has become increasingly focused on the cost and quality of health care. Health care providers are held accountable for their performance and outcomes by third-party payers, patients, legislators, and peers (McBeth & Weydt, 1996, p. 112). Social work and nursing should be very concerned with quality and must make sure quality assurance is an integral component of education and reeducation.

Attention should focus on patient care quality, incorporating efficiency, appropriateness, and effectiveness of care. All health care agencies must improve the quality of the health care they deliver; they can begin by collecting data on admissions, course of stay, variances to the expected course, outcomes (Wood, Bailey, & Tilkemeier, 1992, pp. 55–64), and patient or client satisfaction. This is best accomplished by using a computerized information system. Structure, process, and outcomes all need to be part of a quality assurance evaluation (Auslander & Cohen, 1992, pp. 72, 75–76). After data are examined, problems in health care delivery become evident. The next step then is to plan for change; such planning may include professional development, staffing changes, and departmental training (Shahar, Auslander, & Cohen, 1995, p. 108).

The focus for measuring quality is shifting from processes to outcomes. When measuring quality, appropriateness, efficiency, and effectiveness are important. Outcomes measures are not merely measured at the end of an episode, but also at specific points. Traditional measures of quality have been morbidity, mortality, infection rates, readmission, errors, lengths of stay, complaints, unexpected incidences, and cost. These measures are no longer sufficient, and today quality measurements should include function (activities of daily living, job, family role), health status, activity, mobility, pain, and symptom management (Bower & Falk, 1996, p. 162).

Educating students and professionals in total quality management is one way to improve the quality of health care. In this model, organization-wide continuous improvement requires all persons in the organization to become committed and involved. Three overall objectives used in Cincinnati, Ohio at Bethesda, Inc. were (1) maximizing individual and departmental performance daily by implementation of a system of management of processes; (2) focusing on strategic targets from the very top of the organization to the bottom; and (3) maximizing cooperation and coordination through use of teams that focused on understanding the customer expectations and needs and on improving the processes. Total quality management is not a new educational program for an institution or agency, but a total transformation of the organization (Kaminski, 1992, p. 38). Implementing change and overcoming barriers are important skills to learn.

HEALTH PROMOTION, SELF-CARE, PRIMARY CARE

In communities where a wellness center that focuses on health promotion, self-care, and primary care is not available, programs must be planned, funded, and set up to improve the overall health of the members of the community. Social workers and nurses must learn how to accomplish health promotion for all age groups and for varying ethnic backgrounds and incomes. One way to reduce health care costs is to have consumers assume more responsibility for their health care and do more for themselves. Self-care may include nutrition, exercise, relaxation techniques, stress management, meditation, and other useful techniques.

> Health promotion consists of activities directed toward increasing the level of well being and actualizing the health potential in individuals, families, communities, and society. Primary prevention consists of activities directed toward decreasing the probability of specific illnesses or dysfunctions in individuals, families, and communities, including active protection against necessary stressors. (Pender, 1987, p. 4)

Community screening programs for hypertension, diabetes, depression, and glaucoma; special breast examination clinics and mammography; and health fairs are examples of health promotion activities in the community. Nutrition, exercise and fitness, and stress and self-behavioral management classes are important (Thatcher, 1989, pp. 726–727). Well-baby and child health care should be readily available as should educational programs that include prenatal education; parenting skills; and those that specifically address the unique needs of children, teens, adults, and elderly community members.

Research has shown that a health promotion program for elderly members led to significant improvements in physical health status such as increased flexibility and high density lipoprotein and decreased total cholesterol, blood pressure, resting pulse, weight, and skinfold measurements (Higgins, 1988, p. 710). In another study of 153 healthy women, Hartweg (1993) found these women's healthy self-care activities included balancing rest with meaningful activities; avoiding hazards; solitude; social interactions; healthy eating and eliminating alcohol, caffeine, and chocolate; breathing clean air; self-image care; self-development activities; and routine and preventative health care (pp. 223–225).

HEALTH POLICY/REFORM

Policy courses must include the new service delivery mechanisms and structures and the effect of continually changing policies on health care delivery. Diagnostic related groups, professional standards, cost containment measures, and reimbursability are all important topics that demonstrate the effect of policy on health care delivery. Examination of the current health service delivery systems is very important. Our ever-changing health care system provides powerful and relevant educational examples for students (Strom & Gingerich, 1993, pp. 81, 83–84).

Access is the key to influencing health legislation and policy development. Nurses and social workers have not prioritized sitting at the policy tables in the political arena; we have been reacting instead of initiating health policy and reform. The government is increasingly involved in health care, and nurses (and social workers) should study health policy and carry out health policy-related research (Donley, 1983, pp. 846–847). Access, quality, and cost of health care and direct reimbursement are just some of the issues that they must raise their voices and have a hand in setting the agenda for.

POLITICAL INVOLVEMENT

Although professional organizations in both nursing and social work are politically active on a state and national level, most individuals are not actively involved. For social work and nursing to have a piece of the pie in managed care in the community setting, it is essential they become politically astute and active. With change comes opportunity and nurses and social workers must be there to voice their opinions. For most, learning how to be effective in the political arena is necessary.

Increasingly nurses are becoming politically active on local, regional, state, and federal levels. They are members of boards and on committees and have the opportunity to influence legislation that will determine health care in the future. The political agenda for nursing includes support of reimbursement for advanced practice nurses, assessment and evaluation of intervention and treatment through research, promotion of innovative care delivery in nursing centers, and publication of quality and outcome data. Health care for all at a reasonable cost is most likely to happen with primary care in the community, supplemented by hospitals and other institutions. Nurses and social workers must help consumers to become informed participants in their own care (DeBack & Cohen, 1996, pp. 6–7). More individual social workers and nurses need to become politically involved.

ETHICS

As the argument continues about whether health care is a right or a privilege, managed care is creating ethical dilemmas undreamed of during the federal War on Poverty of the 1960s and early 1970s or the New Deal of the 1930s (when an early attempt was made and defeated to mandate health care for all). From an ethic of do anything possible and a high technology approach to care, we have moved rapidly to rationing of care. Coming from a stance of justice laid in the cornerstone of each profession during the 19th century, nursing and social work find themselves in a quagmire as they survey the current landscape of health care. Social workers and nurses created systems to assure access to basic care for immigrants, school children, workers, tenement dwellers, and rural and city residents. Those systems slowly unravelled under the pressures of escalating health care costs, decreasing numbers of Americans with health insurance, and a shift to managed care. Control of decisions about health care is slipping from the hands of consumers and their health care providers into those of executives of large for-profit care conglomerates and third-party payers. Increasingly these giants of the health care industry are joining forces through managed care systems. Although managed care is not new, nor is it inherently evil, as Zoloth-Dorfman and Rubin pointed out, for-profit plans in particular "have been criticized as threatening to weaken or displace the professional commitments to beneficence and nonmaleficence that are the foundation of the therapeutic relationship'' (1995, p. 341). These authors went on to ask: "How can physicians, nurses and other healthcare providers who work in managed care be assured that their professional integrity will not be compromised by their being compelled to participate in care that they deem to be substandard'' (Zoloth-Dorfman & Rubin, 1995, p. 341)?

In an analysis of proposals for a "just management of scarce health care resources," the authors endorsed policies placing limits on the public finance of health services that are nonbasic, advocated using a medical benefit standard to distribute health care resources among individuals, and endorsed equality as the goal in providing basic health care (Jecker & Pearlman, 1992, pp. 91–92). A number of court cases have challenged the ethics of managed care systems denying patients access to services (Davis, 1995). If social workers and nurses are absent when decisions are made about funding technology, distribution of health care resources, and principles of justice in access to basic health care, they will be depriving decision makers of the opinions of the largest collective group of health care professionals. Moreover, it might be argued that they are abdicating, by their silence, their responsibility as professionals who practice under codes of ethics.

On a case-by-case basis, professionals are confronted with ethical dilemmas about access to basic health care or to health care resources. When one can put names and faces to these dilemmas, personal ethos is challenged directly. As managed care systems, particularly those that are for-profit[1], become more ruthless in their pursuit of the bottom line, providers are forced into choices that hinder their ability to care about and for patients. Some managed care systems even offer financial incentives to providers to limit care (Council on Ethical and Judicial Affairs of the American Medical Association, 1995). This is particularly troublesome when we consider patient problems that require long-term care such as mental illness (Iglehart, 1996; Stern, 1993) and chronic conditions. When there are no safeguards to assure that limits on services occur only when those services are not essential to the well-being of patients, providers are placed in ethically precarious positions.

As the historic defenders of the disenfranchised of society—the poor; children; women; elderly persons; persons with physical and developmental disabilities; persons with social diseases such as tuberculosis, sexually transmitted diseases and AIDS; and persons with mental illness—

---

[1]As Christensen (1995) pointed out, managed care is not a singular entity. All managed care organizations struggle with providing all necessary care while controlling costs.

nurses and social workers find themselves posturing for new defenses. Over the past decade, in the name of deinstitutionalization, mental hospitals, orphanages, county poor farms, state hospitals for persons with mental retardation, and municipal homes for elderly persons have been emptied, leaving these individuals, in many cases, not only defenseless but also homeless. Now they are being herded under the managed care blanket in the guise of better care than Medicare (or Medicaid and other publicly funded health and social services programs). Critics of managed care organizations have argued that "dissolution of existing, in many instances venerable, social service/mental health agencies has seriously undermined treatment for the poor, for racial and ethnic minorities, and for the seriously disturbed . . . "(Schamess, 1996, p. 211). Many of these individuals are high risk, high utilization patients, making them unattractive to the very systems currently courting their business through publicly funded programs, leaving their care providers somewhere between the proverbial rock and hard place in advocating for needed services and being forced to watch the bottom line. Care providers are also being forced to care more than ever about the records they keep on clients and the relationship between such records and future access to care.

The technological revolution means that data can be created, stored, and communicated by a variety of means and to an audience as small or as large as the creator of those data might wish or feel is appropriate. The adoption by managed care organizations of electronic means to create patient records means that those data are available in a way not possible with traditional paper files. This ability has created ethical issues about confidentiality of information (Davidson & Davidson, 1996; Gostin et al., 1993). Theoretically, data about patients could be accessed by payers, employers, managers of employee benefit packages, virtually anyone with a computer and the codes necessary for entry into the database. As we consider new incentives for patients to change their lifestyles, one can envision an Orwellian scenario of control over personal choice.

Imbedded in the concept of health maintenance organizations, the parents of managed care systems, is a belief that over time, maintaining health (disease prevention and health promotion) is cheaper than treating illness. When individuals choose lifestyles that damage their health, ultimately we all pay the bill for the care they then require (Morreim, 1995). As part of the ethic of caring within managed care systems nurses and social workers are challenged to "ensure that all those with an important stake in the health care system—payers, providers, and patients alike—use its resources . . . wisely" (Morreim, 1995, p. 11). The question is how to do this without sinking into a blame-the-victim mentality. As health care providers best prepared to work with individuals, families, groups, and

communities, nurses and social workers can create models of health promotion and disease prevention that will empower patients with a "greater
measure of control over their health care" (Morreim, 1995, p. 11). Social
workers and nurses demonstrated their ability to do this in the 19th and
early 20th century with prenatal care, immunizations, and other preventive
and early intervention measures and are capable of doing so again. Some
of the models presented in the preceding chapters speak to the feasibility
of empowering those to whom care is provided.

Some health care professionals, in their efforts to protect patients from
managed care organizations, have adopted radical responses, including
appealing decisions not to cover an intervention, trying to "game the
system," or providing care out of their own pockets (Howe, 1995, p. 290).
Howe suggested adopting the perspective of philosopher Jean-Francois
Lyotard by suspending our judgment about managed care systems and
being open to their potential. Such an attitude might provide, in Howe's
words, a view of managed care systems "from a transcendent, more
insightful perspective" (1995, p. 300). It might also help create a sense
of community and decrease the stresses: "Both managed-care reviewers
and care providers seek to help patients; both hurt because their resources
have to be limited" (Howe, 1995, p. 301).

As members of professions guided by codes of ethics, nurses and social
workers have those ethics to guide their practices in this increasingly
inhumane, so-called system. Social work's code (National Association of
Social Workers, 1993) is specific in its principles addressing service and
ethical responsibilities to clients: "The social worker should regard as
primary the service obligation of the social work profession. . . . The social
worker's primary responsibility is to clients" (p. 1). Nursing's code is
more general: "The nurse provides services with respect for human dignity
and the uniqueness of the client, unrestricted by considerations of social
or economic status, personal attributes, or the nature of health problems. . . . The nurse acts to safeguard the client and the public when health
care and safety are affected by the incompetent, unethical, or illegal
practice of any person (American Nurses Association, 1985, p. 1). The
ethics committee of the National Association of Social Workers has determined that social workers must consider and judge the ethics of programs
and institutions, as well as those of individual practitioners (Sabin, 1994).
Likewise, nurses must concern themselves with the "ethics of institutional
and social obligations as well as obligations to individual patients" (Aroskar, 1994, p. 11). In the spirit of our founders, notably Florence Nightingale and Jane Addams, we cannot abdicate "the development of healing
environments as a nursing responsibility and nurses' obligations to protect
patient confidentiality" (Aroskar, 1994, p. 11) and the "major objective of

social work practice . . . to develop and strengthen communally supported services and to enable participants to make use of social resources available to them'' (Specht & Courtney, 1994, p. 171).

The model of collaboration we have proposed, drawn from the literature and from our participants, is congruent with these ethical tenets and obligates us to continue the quest for the best in practice, education, and research.

RESEARCH

Research, now increasingly and necessarily interdisciplinary, is integrating new technologies. Technological innovations enable practitioners to collect assessment and intervention data, store these data for outcome studies, examine facets of their practice, and study the human response patterns of their patients.

There are three major concerns in research in managed health and behavioral health care systems: initial assessment and goal-setting, calibrating the processes of interventions in the community, and outcome evaluations. These three areas mirror both the practice and research processes. The strengths and stresses inherent in the interdisciplinary model we have proposed will be played out in research efforts because every step must be jointly designed and implemented by the social workers and nurses on the collaborative team.

INITIAL ASSESSMENT AND GOAL SETTING

In previous chapters the point has been made that it is essential to set clear and measurable initial goals for all cases and projects. Nursing has well-conceptualized and extensive intervention protocols, sometimes called care or critical pathways. Social work does not have such protocols and, although they are in the beginning of developing them in certain areas such as home health care, this lack severely limits initial clear goal setting against which to evaluate the outcomes of social work interventions. What is recommended here is joint social work-nursing protocol development, on a case-by-case or situation-specific basis, in the collaborative Biopsychosocial Individual and System Intervention Model (BISIM) proposed previously.

Not only would joint initial assessment and goal and protocol setting objectify benchmarks for outcome evaluations, but it would cut down on the use of fuzzy and often inappropriate preexisting assessment and diagnostic tools discussed in chapter 7. If initial goals and objectives are set in measurable terms by the social worker–nurse collaborative team, then they are owned by the team, and outcome evaluation will be a cooperative and collaborative endeavor, not a competitive one. The research model being suggested is widely described currently as scientist-practitioner (Bronson, 1994; Dangel, 1994; Hudson & Nurius, 1994) or practitioner-researcher (Hess & Mullen, 1995; Mailick, King, Donnelly, & Euster, 1995).

CALIBRATING THE PROCESSES OF INTERVENTIONS IN THE COMMUNITY

The process of intervention must be constantly measured. Each BISIM nurse-social work collaborative team must develop a way to note or scale processes and progress in a way that enables measurement at some outcome point. One useful process and outcome measuring technique is goal attainment scaling, the parsimony and validity of which make it particularly useful in health and behavioral health settings (Kiresuk, Smith, & Cardillo, 1994).

OUTCOME EVALUATIONS

Outcome evaluations are the rage in health and behavioral health care services delivery. This is appropriate, given managed health care's dual focus on efficiency and effectiveness. However, a recent newspaper headline questioned, "is research being 'managed' out of existence?" This article points out that results of new treatments, even those that would benefit vast majorities of individuals and groups, are "regarded as trade secrets and knowledge is hoarded" (Gordon, 1996, p. D2). It must be noted that managed care companies are currently handling their treatment and interventions protocols as proprietary and not for dissemination.

If information in the aggregate is not available to researchers, research efforts are severely curtailed. Nurse–social work teams must not let this happen. All of the team's efforts must have outcome evaluations so that the practice may be improved on a team-wide basis across targeted individuals and groups. These efforts will be greatly enhanced by computer technology, with its immense storage, retrieval, analysis, depicting, and reporting capacities (Nurius & Hudson, 1988).

Team processes and outcomes must be consistently and constantly evaluated. There must be an openness about data gathering and analysis throughout the interdisciplinary nurse–social work team. In addition to evaluating the results of specific team interventions, some other suggested areas for collaborative team research are combined quantitative and qualitative studies of documenting what families and communities are doing for themselves (strengths to be worked with and built on); needed policy supports (Freeman, 1996); administrative and management issues in community health and behavioral health care delivery; role relationships and their enhancement in interdisciplinary teams; and evaluations of innovative interventions for individuals, families, groups, communities, and organizations in community settings.

CONCLUDING THOUGHTS, COMMON VOICES

The central mission of both nursing and social work began in the community at the end of the 19th century. As we hang on the cusp of the 20th century, it returns to the community. Nurses and social workers are the experts on the community and its problems. The chaos in the health care delivery system created by the stampede to managed care and its offspring has sent both nursing and social work reeling. The environment for health care delivery may never be as institution-based as it has been in this century. The response of professional caregivers can take many forms. If they adopt a position of reacting to the chaos by clinging to the past and insisting that they can only practice from an institutional base, they will miss opportunities as stellar as they were at the end of the 19th century. If they choose to be proactive, discarding or at least reexamining their fascination with institution-based models of care delivery, they are free to dream ways to deliver care that do not yet exist.

The BISIM intervention model is neither institution based nor restrictive in its utility as a conceptual base from which to create care delivery systems designed to respond to the needs of individuals, families, groups, and communities. Social workers and nurses have the skills and knowledge to collaborate to improve service delivery to consumers whoever they might be, and they might be communities, companies, schools, or neighborhoods, as well as individuals, families, and groups. Just as social workers and nurses engaged in preventive education with new immigrants, school children, cannery workers, stone masons, pregnant women, and children during the infancy of public health nursing, medical social work, and collaboration between social workers and nurses in settlement houses, they can create services to meet the health and social services needs for the 21st century and plan and carry out research designed to measure outcomes.[2] In so doing, they can also create new educational models for

---

[2]Mary Breckinridge, founder of the Frontier Nursing Service; Lillian Wald and Lina Rogers, the founders of school nursing and pioneers in settlement house work; Jane Addams; and many more of our foremothers and forefathers in nursing and social work collected data and demonstrated that the models of care delivery they had created made a difference in outcomes.

students so that they learn collaboration along the road to professional preparation.

"Social workers and nurses should take the helm in developing the new leadership skills needed to implement major change, and the management of process, and how not only to help each other fit into the new delivery system but assist the patient(s) to also know what changed and how and where they access the system" (study participant, 1996).

In an address to Vassar students in 1915, Lillian Wald said the following: "Women and with them at times far-seeing men, prophetic because they knew the movements of the past, have helped to open up opportunities in the professions, not as special privileges, but to endow woman (and man) that (their) natural gifts might come to full fruition, and not for . . . the individual, but for all—womankind and mankind—to serve the community" (p. 82). Nurses and social workers must seize the opportunities. If they don't, they face an uncertain and perhaps disastrous demise.

REFERENCES

American Nurses Association. (1985). *Code for nurses with interpretive statements.* Kansas City, MO: Author.

Aroskar, M. A. (1994). Ethics in nursing and health care reform: Back to the future? *Hastings Center Report, 24*(3), 11–12.

Auslander, G. K., & Cohen, M. E. (1992). The role of computerized information systems in quality assurance in hospital social work departments. *Social Work in Health Care, 18*(10), 71–92.

Berkman, B. (1996). The emerging health care world: Implications for social work practice and education. *Social Work, 41,* 541–551.

Berkman, B., Shearer, S., Simmons, W. J., White, M., Robinson, M., Sampson, S., Holmes, W., Allison, D., & Thomson, J. A. (1996). Ambulatory elderly patients of primary care physicians: Functional, psychosocial and environment predictors of need for social work care management. *Social Work in Health Care, 22*(3), 1–20.

Bower, K. A., & Falk, C. D. (1996). Case management as a response to quality, cost, and access imperatives. In E. L. Cohen (Ed.), *Nurse case management in the 21st century* (pp. 161–167). St. Louis: Mosby.

Bronson, D. E. (1994). Is a scientist-practitioner model appropriate for direct social work practice? No. In W. W. Hudson & P. S. Nurius (Eds.), *Controversial issues in social work research* (pp. 79–86). Boston: Allyn and Bacon.

Christensen, K. T. (1995). Ethically important distinctions among managed care organizations. *Journal of Law, Medicine, & Ethics, 23,* 223–229.

Council on Ethical and Judicial Affairs, American Medical Association. (1995). Ethical issues in managed care. *Journal of the American Medical Association, 273,* 330–335.

Dangel, R. F. (1994). Is a scientist-practitioner model appropriate for direct social work practice? Yes. In W. W. Hudson & P. S. Nurius (Eds.), *Controversial issues in social work research* (pp. 75–81). Boston: Allyn and Bacon.

Davidson, J. R., & Davidson, T. (1996). Confidentiality and managed care: Ethical and legal considerations. *Health & Social Work, 21*, 208–215.

Davis, D. S. (1995). Legal trends in bioethics. *Journal of Clinical Ethics, 6*, 380–384.

Davis, V. (1996). Staff development for nurse case management. In E. L. Cohen (Ed.), *Nurse case management in the 21st century* (pp. 189–201). St. Louis: Mosby.

DeBack, V., & Cohen, E. (1996). The new practice environment. In E. L. Cohen (Ed.), *Nurse case management in the 21st century* (pp. 3–9). St. Louis: Mosby.

Donley, S. M. (1983). Nursing and the politics of health. In N. L. Chaska (Ed.), *The nursing profession: A time to speak* (pp. 844–857). New York: McGraw-Hill.

Donner, S. (1996). Field work crisis: Dilemmas, dangers and opportunities. *Smith College Studies in Social Work, 66*, 317–331.

Freeman, E. M. (1996). Welfare reforms and services for children and families: Setting a new practice, research, and policy agenda. *Social Work, 41*, 521–532.

Gordon, S. (1996, October 13). Is research being "managed" out of existence? *Boston Globe*, pp. D1–2.

Gostin, L. O., Turek-Brezina, J., Powers, M., Kozloff, R., Faden, R., & Steinauer, D. D. (1993). Privacy and security of personal information in a new health care system. *Journal of the American Medical Association, 270*, 2487–2493.

Hartweg, D. L. (1993). Self-care actions of healthy middle-aged women to promote well-being. *Nursing Research, 42*(4), 221–226.

Hess, P. McC., & Mullen, E. J. (Eds.). (1995). *Practitioner-researcher partnerships. Building knowledge from, in, and for practice.* Washington: NASW Press.

Hey, M. (1993). Nursing's renaissance: An innovative continuum of care takes nurses back to their roots. *Health Progress, October*, 26–32.

Higgins, P. G. (1988). Biometric outcome of a geriatric health promotion programme. *Journal of Advanced Nursing, 13*, 710–715.

Howe, E. G. (1995). Managed care: "New moves," moral uncertainty, and a radical attitude. *Journal of Clinical Ethics, 6*(4), 290–305.

Hudson, W. W., & Nurius, P. S. (1994). *Controversial issues in social work research.* Boston: Allyn and Bacon.

Iglehart, J. K. (1996). Managed care and mental health. *New England Journal of Medicine, 334*, 131–135.

Jecker, N. S., & Pearlman, R. A. (1992). An ethical framework for rationing health care. *Journal of Medicine and Philosophy, 17*, 79–96.

Kaminski, G. (1992). Total quality management at Bethesda, Inc. Journal for Healthcare Quality: *Promoting Excellence in Healthcare, 14*(6), 38–53.

Kiresuk, T. J., Smith, A., & Cardillo, J. E. (1994). *Goal attainment scaling: Applications, theory, and measurement.* Hillsdale, NJ: Lawrence Erlbaum.

Kurtz, L. F., Bagarozzi, D. A., & Pollane, L. P. (1984). Case management in mental health. *Health and Social Work*, 201–211.

Mailick, M. D., King, M. A., Donnelly, J., & Euster, S. (1995). Practitioners as researchers. Development of a collaborative model. In P. McC. Hess & E. J. Mullen (Eds.), *Practitioner-researcher partnerships. Building knowledge from, in, and for practice* (pp. 89–205). Washington: NASW Press.

Malloy, C. (1995). Health care reform and implications for nursing. *Journal of Health Care Practice, 7*(4), 76–85.

McBeth, A., & Weydt, A. (1996). Innovative delivery systems: Freedom, trust, caring. In E. L. Cohen (Ed.), *Nurse case management in the 21st century* (pp. 105–116). St. Louis: Mosby.

McNutt, J. G. (1995). The macro practice curriculum in graduate social work education: Results of a national study. *Administration in Social Work, 19*(3), 59–74.

Morreim, E. H. (1995). Lifestyles of the risky and infamous: From managed care to managed lives. *Hastings Center Report, 25*(5), 5–11.

National Association of Social Workers. (1993). *Code of ethics of the National Association of Social Workers.* Washington, DC: Author.

Nurius, P. S., & Hudson, W. W. (1988). Computer-based practice: Future dream or current technology? *Social Work, 33,* 357–362.

Pender, N. J. (1987). *Health promotion in nursing practice* (2nd ed.). Norwalk, CT: Appleton & Lange.

Poole, D. (1995). Shaking the kaleidoscope. *Health and Social Work, 20*(3), 163–165.

Ramay, J. (1996, July/August). Why integrate? A behavioral perspective. *Behavioral Health Management,* pp. 20–21.

Sabin, J. E. (1994). Caring about patients and caring about money: The American Psychiatric Association code of ethics meets managed care. *Behavioral Sciences and the Law, 12,* 317–330.

Salzman, P. (1996, July/August). Integrating community services for prevention. *Behavioral Health Management,* pp. 9–13.

Schamess, G. (1996). Who profits and who benefits from managed mental health care? *Smith College Studies in Social Work, 66,* 209–220.

Shahar, I. B., Auslander, G., & Cohen, M. (1995). Utilizing date to improve practice in hospital social work: A case study. *Social Work in Health Care, 20*(3), 99–111.

Shamansky, S. L. (1995). A longer-than-usual editorial about population-based managed care. *Public Health Nursing, 12,* 211–212.

Smith, J. R., & Shiner, P. M. (1996). Transforming nursing practice: Acute to community care. *Home Health Care Management, 8*(5), 32–39.

Specht, H., & Courtney, M. E. (1994). *Unfaithful angels: How social work has abandoned its mission.* New York: Free Press.

Stern, S. (1993). Managed care, brief therapy, and therapeutic integrity. *Psychotherapy, 30,* 162–175.

Strom, K., & Gingerich, W. J. (1993). Educating students for the new market realities. *Journal of Social Work Education, 29,* 78–87.

Thatcher, R. M. (1989). Community support: Promoting health and self care. *Nursing Clinics of North America, 24,* 725–731.

Wald, L. (1989). New aspects of old social responsibilities. Address to Vassar students (1915), reprinted in C. Coss (Ed.), *Lillian D. Wald progressive activist* (pp. 76–84). New York: Feminist Press.

Wood, R. G., Bailey, N. O., & Tilkemeier, D. (1992). Managed care: The missing link in quality improvement. *Journal of Nursing Care Quality, 6*(4), 55–65.

Zoloth-Dorfman, L., & Rubin, S. (1995). The patient as commodity: Managed care and the question of ethics. *Journal of Clinical Ethics, 6,* 339–357.

Appendix: Design of the Nurse–Social Worker Collaboration Study

We prepared for our study by examining feminist methods of research.[1] Reinharz (1979, 1981, 1992) has written extensively about women as researchers and research by and about women. Reinharz wrote that one of the differences between mainstream sociological research models and the alternative method (new paradigm) she proposed is an interest in the latter in "the meaningfulness of research findings to the scholarly and user communities" and in "generating concepts in vivo, in the field itself" (1979, pp. 11–12). She suggested that we might study "natural events encased in their ongoing contexts" and elicit "feelings, behavior, thoughts, insights, and actions as witnessed or experienced" (1979, pp. 14–15). Reinharz (1981) also underscored the necessity for a supportive environment to conduct research in the alternative method.

In an extensive review of the literature on interviewing as a preferred method for feminist research, Reinharz (1992) explored the positive attributes of open-ended or semistructured interviews through the eyes of feminist researchers. She concluded that this method allows feminist researchers to create "important new ways of seeing the world. By listening to women speak, understanding women's membership in particular social systems, and establishing the distribution of phenomena accessible only through sensitive interviewing, feminist interview researchers have uncovered previously neglected or misunderstood worlds of experience" (p. 44).

We were guided also by the work of other feminist researchers (Belenky, Clinchy, Goldberger, & Tarule, 1986; Finch, 1984; Fornow & Cook,

---

[1]Veeder noted in *Women's Decision-Making* (1992) that: "I do not like the term *feminist research* since the research generated under a feminist label runs the considerable risk of being seen as possessing lesser status both in academia and the wider society, given the focus on women (who have lesser status in society simply based on gender)" (note 1, p. 33). We have used the term to identify a viewpoint that diverges significantly from that of the male majority of social science researchers.

1991; Gilligan, 1980, 1982; Gilligan, Lyons, & Hanmer, 1989; Gilligan, Ward, & Taylor, 1988; Gluck, 1979; Graham, 1984; Harding, 1987; Nielsen, 1990; Patai, 1983; Riessman, 1990; Roberts, 1990; Stern & Pyles, 1985; Tuana, 1989). Most importantly, we wanted to hear the voices of our participants as they shared their views of the challenges facing social workers and nurses, current models for collaboration, and their dreams. Because we are all social workers or nurses, we brought ourselves as instruments to the research process, along with our own biases, experiences, and dreams. We were, in Reinharz's words, "involved (and had a) sense of commitment, participation, and sharing of fate" with the participants (1979, pp. 14–15).

STUDY FORMULATION

We designed the study with the foregoing as premises for the research, as well as guideposts so that we would be true to our participants' voices. The major questions we explored were

- What is the history of collaboration between social workers and nursing in a variety of agencies and institutions?
- What are the pluses and minuses in the ways in which social workers and nurses interact; how can social workers and nurses evaluate the outcomes of their practices or interventions?
- What might an ideal system of collaboration look like?
- What opportunities might managed care or a system of capitation offer for nurses, social workers, and their clients for access to care, a holistic approach to care, health promotion and disease prevention, and integration of alternative or complementary therapies?
- What new opportunities might there be for collaboration between these two professions?

The most appropriate method to use to answer the study questions was feminist interview research. Anticipating that many, if not most, of the participants would be women, we also recognized the congruence between this method and achieving "the active involvement of their (feminists') respondents in the construction of data about their lives (Graham, 1984, p. 112).

THE INTERVIEW

Each participant was interviewed at the place of work,[2] and the approximately 30-minute interview was audiotaped. We facilitated the interview

---

[2]Reinharz (1979) suggested that "data gathering in natural settings can alert the researcher to the presence of information that is already available in the setting such as archives, reports, ... "

process by speaking with each participant on the telephone prior to the interview and by sending information about the study in a letter requesting participation (see Exhibit 1). We offered and sent the study questions to each participant who requested them. Each of the seven questions was open ended and we asked at the end of the interview whether there were any other important areas we had not covered in the seven questions or any other information the participant wished to share with us (see Exhibit 2).

In preparation for the interviews, beside creating, discussing, and then revising the questions that would guide our interviews, we also created an introduction to the study that we would both send to each participant and use by way of introduction at the beginning of each interview to focus the discussion (see Exhibit 3). We all participated in a training session led by our social work team member, then discussed the role playing used as part of the training technique, making suggestions about how to conduct interviews (see Exhibit 4). During these sessions, we investigated our own "previous experiences, intentions, hopes and preju-dices to try to understand what (we) were bringing to the study" (Reinharz, 1979, p. 13). After several interviews, we met as a research team, listened to the tapes of the interviews, and made suggestions for improvement of the interview technique and refinement of the questions. We also began to analyze the data for meaningful patterns (see Exhibit 5). The group meetings served to move the project forward and also created for each of us the "supportive environment" Reinharz urged as necessary to re-search in the new paradigm (1981, p. 426).

We wrote field notes after each interview to capture the context and nonverbal content of the interview that would be lost on the audiotape. We checked and listened to each tape as soon as possible after the interview in preparation for the next. Sometimes we had the opportunity to interview the social worker and the nurse at a particular setting on the same day or in a close time framework so that we could build from one interview onto the other. If that was not possible, we could review our field notes and the tape of the first interview before the second at that setting. We also did member checking with the participants as themes emerged, asking if they had the same perceptions of the opportunities, pluses, and minuses of collaboration.

Our participants, the scholarly and user community, were "addressed and engaged" (Reinharz, 1979, pp. 14–15). They provided us with feed-back as to the completeness, plausibility, illustrativeness, and understand-ing with which we viewed the interview data and our responsiveness to their experiences (Reinharz, 1979, pp. 14–15).

THE SAMPLE

In preparation for soliciting participants, we generated a list of possible agencies and institutions employing both social workers and nurses. We included large teaching institutions, community agencies, those offering primarily inpatient care, those totally community based, and those with a continuum of care. The study sites also include those offering both specialty and generalist health care services, ambulatory care, home care, acute, subacute and long-term care, and multidimensional services for special groups such as women using substances during pregnancy and children with developmental delays (see Exhibit 6 for profiles of agencies and institutions). Once we had identified potential study sites representing as wide a variety of health and social services wherein both nurses and social workers might have at least the opportunity to collaborate, we began to identify persons in leadership positions in those settings. In so doing, we constructed a purposive sample by consciously seeking the directors of social services or social work and the vice presidents, clinical directors, or directors of nursing or patient care services. Most importantly, the person holding the position had to be credentialed as a social worker or nurse. Two nurses held the position of president or chief executive officer of the agency or institution. The social worker–nurse teams who practice in two focused models of collaboration were included because they demonstrate what is possible when these two professions have the opportunity to interact in the best interests of those for whom they care with special needs. Some agencies and institutions have very flat or decentralized management. In these cases, we interviewed nurse–social work teams at the same level on the organizational chart or comparable positions in power and decision making about patient care. In two agencies, we interviewed two social workers and one nurse and in one we interviewed two nurses, one of whom is also a social worker, and one social worker. Many of our participants had practiced in a variety of settings and could offer rich data about those settings and the opportunities for collaboration.

The sample consisted of 16 nurses, 16 social workers, and one person who is a social worker and a nurse from 16 different agencies (see Exhibit 7 for profile of participants, Exhibit 8 for a profile of the participants and their agencies, and Exhibit 9 for the consent form). Most of the participants are women, reflecting the preponderance of women in both professions. From a historic perspective, the sample reflects not only what is in the 1990s, but what was in the 1890s when the collaboration between these two professions developed in the settlement houses.

ANALYSIS OF THE INTERVIEW DATA

As we completed each interview, we listened to the tape before proceeding with the next. Reinharz (1979) suggested that in the alternative model, data analysis occur during rather than after data collection is complete, and that the researcher rely on inductive rather than deductive logic. We met as a group to share interviews and discuss their content and emerging themes. We used content-analysis to review and analyze the qualitative data from the interviews. We then began to create "gestalts and meaningful patterns" (Reinharz, 1979, pp. 14–15) from the information. Each team member listened to the tapes of the interviews she had conducted and typed notes from the tape, including direct quotes from the participants to be used in telling the story of collaboration. The emphasis, always, was on exploring in depth and understanding the participants' views of collaboration between the two professions; their stories of successful and not so successful models of collaboration; analysis of the pluses and minuses of such collaboration, and what we might do about the latter; and their vision of the present and the future opportunities for such collaboration under managed care, capitation, and whatever is to follow.

After collecting and analyzing the data, we then did an extensive literature search. The goal of this search was to compare and contrast themes emerging from the data with the extant literature on those themes. Ultimately this led to theory building about the nature of and potential for collaborative relationships between social workers and nurses in this time of chaos and for the 21st century. Chapter 4 explores the themes that emerged from the data.

REFERENCES

Belenky, M. F., Clinchy, B., Goldberger, N. R., & Tarule, J. M. (1986). *Women's ways of knowing: The development of self, voice, and mind.* New York: Basic Books.

Finch, J. (1984). "It's great to have someone to talk to": The ethics and politics of interviewing women. In C. Bell & H. Roberts (Eds.), *Social researching: Politics, problems, practice* (pp. 70–87). London: Routledge & Kegan Paul.

Fornow, M. M., & Cook, J. A. (Eds.). (1991). *Beyond methodology: Feminist scholarship as lived research.* Indianapolis, IN: Indiana University Press.

Gilligan, C. (1980). Restoring the missing text of women's development to life cycle theories. In D. G. McGuigan (Ed)., *Women's lives: New theory, research and policy* (pp. 17–33). Ann Arbor, MI: University of Michigan Center for Continuing Education of Women.

Gilligan, C. (1982). *In a different voice: Psychological theory and women's development.* Cambridge, MA: Harvard University Press.

Gilligan, C., Lyons, N., & Hanmer, T. J. (1989). *Making connections: The relational worlds of adolescent girls at Emma Willard School.* Troy, NY: Emma Willard School.

Gilligan, C., Ward, J. V., & Taylor, J. M. (Eds.). (1988). *Mapping the moral domain.* Cambridge, MA: Harvard University Press.

Gluck, S. (1979). What's so special about women? Women's oral history. *Frontiers, 2,* 3–11.

Graham, H. (1984). Surveying through stories. In C. Bell & H. Roberts (Eds.), *Social researching: Politics, problems, practice* (pp. 104–124). London: Routledge & Kegan Paul.

Harding, S. (Ed.). (1987). *Feminism & methodology.* Indianapolis, IN: Indiana University Press.

Nielsen, J. M. (Ed.). (1990). *Feminist research methods.* Boulder, CO: Westview Press.

Patai, D. (1983). Beyond defensiveness: Feminist research strategies. *Women's Studies International Forum, 6,* 177–189.

Reinharz, S. (1979). *On becoming a social scientist.* San Francisco: Jossey-Bass.

Reinharz, S. (1981). Implementing new paradigm research: A model for training and practice. In P. Reason & J. Rowan, *A sourcebook of new paradigm research* (pp. 415–436). New York: John Wiley.

Reinharz, S. (1992). *Feminist methods in social research.* New York: Oxford University Press.

Riessman, C. K. (1990). *Divorce talk: Women and men make sense of personal relationships.* New Brunswick, NJ: Rutgers University Press.

Roberts, H. (Ed.). (1990). *Doing feminist research.* New York: Routledge.

Stern, P., & Poyles, S. H. (1985). Using grounded theory methodology to study women's culturally based decisions about health. *Health Care for Women International, 6,* (1–3), 1–24.

Tuana, N. (1989). *Feminism & science.* Bloomington, IN: Indiana University Press.

EXHIBIT 1   Letter Requesting Participation in the Study

BOSTON COLLEGE
CHESTNUT HILL, MASSACHUSETTS 02167

School of Nursing
Tel. (617) 552-4252
FAX (617) 552-0745
email HAWKINSJ@HERMES.BC.EDU

October 15, 1995

Dear

We, two nurses and one social worker, are collaborating on a new book which is under contract with Springer Publishing. The title of the book is *Managed Care: Social Work and Nursing Uniting to Take Charge in the Community. A Model of Collaboration, Coordination, and Accountability.*

We are writing to invite you to participate in an exciting project to explore the roles and the future of our two professions, nursing and social work, in the evolving managed care environment. These times of chaos are an unprecedented opportunity for nursing and social work, historically linked so closely in the community, to work together and to create new systems of care within the managed care framework as the latter changes and evolves. As care returns to the community and becomes less setting focused and driven, we can seize the opportunity to evolve together and capitalize on our common strengths and our important differences. A major issue in managed care is how these two professions do and will interact.

As background and foreground for this important and exciting book we are surveying a small group of social workers and nurses in top decision-making positions in a range of health and behavioral health settings. We hope that you will agree to be interviewed.

The format for our study is structured interviews. The interview is designed to last no more than 30 minutes. Interviews will be audiotaped so that the interviewers can capture the entire interview without disrupting it for note taking. We will be conducting the interviews with the assistance of three graduate students. The end product of this effort will be a book under contract with Springer Publishing.

Within a few days of your receiving this letter, one of our interviewers will telephone you to set up an appointment time convenient to you. The interview will be conducted at your site.

We thank you in advance for assisting us in this collaborative project concerning the future of social work–nursing practice in managed care systems.

Sincerely,

Joellen W. Hawkins, RNC, Ph.D., FAAN
Professor

Nancy W. Veeder, Ph.D., LICSW
Associate Professor, Graduate School of Social Work

Carole W. Pearce, RNC, Ph.D.
Assistant Professor, University of Massachusetts Lowell

EXHIBIT 2   Questions for Study of Social Workers and Nurses in Managed Care Systems

1. Please trace the beginning and evolution of nursing–social work interactions in your managed care system.
2. What do you see as the major pluses in the way nurses and social workers interact?
3. In every interaction there are always some pluses and minuses. Can you describe any problems in interactions between nurses and social workers?
4. Do you have some ideas about how both nurses and social workers could evaluate the outcomes of their practice or interventions?
5. Do you envision more opportunities for direct access by the client to a variety of services under managed care? If so, how?
6. If you could design an ideal system for nursing and social work collaboration in managed care settings of the future, what would it look like?

   a. Can we build a model in managed care that is true health promotion and holistic in its approach, cost effective , and truly interdisciplinary? If so, how?
   b. Do you envision integration of alternative healers, strategies and so on in a managed care model, especially recognizing the multi-cultural nature of society? If so, how?

[Be specific on the planning]

7. Which opportunities, currently untapped, do you see for both nurses and social workers in managed care systems in the future?
8. Are there any other important areas not covered by the previous questions that you would like to share with us?

EXHIBIT 3   "Introduction to the Study" (Statement Read to Each Participant)

These times of chaos are an unprecedented opportunity for nursing and social work, historically linked so closely in the community, to work together and to create new systems of care within the managed care framework as the latter changes and evolves. From a base of evolution together as professions for women primarily in the community, nursing and social work then diverged, driven by the social welfare system and the medical model and its megasystem. As care returns to the community and becomes less setting focused and driven, we can seize the opportunity to evolve together and capitalize on our common strengths and our important differences. A major issue in managed care is how these two professions do and will interact.

We appreciate your taking time to help us explore some of the issues in this interface and to share with us your ideas as you view your profession in the evolving system of care, whatever that may be.

EXHIBIT 4   Protocols for Interview Schedule

INTRODUCTION TO THE STUDY (TO BE READ, VERBATIM, TO EACH STUDY PARTICIPANT)

These times of chaos are an unprecedented opportunity for nursing and social work, historically linked so closely in the community, to work together and to create new systems of care within the managed care framework as the latter changes and evolves. From a base of evolution together as professions for women primarily in the community, nursing and social work then diverged, driven by the social welfare system and the medical model and its megasystem. As care returns to the community and becomes less setting-focused and driven, we can seize the opportunity to evolve together and capitalize on our common strengths and our important differences. A major issue in managed care is how these two professions do and will interact.

We appreciate your taking time to help us explore some of the issues in this interface and to share with us your ideas as you view your profession in the evolving system of care, whatever that may be.

QUESTIONS

1.   Probe for specific examples of these previous interactions and changes in them as they evolved.
2.   Probe for as many pluses as possible.
3.   Probe for as many minuses as possible.
4.   Probe for specific outcome evaluations and techniques.
5.   Probe for specific and many direct-access-to-services opportunities.
6.   Probe for specifics in many areas of ideal nursing–social work collaboration in managed care settings.
6a.   Be specific about "how" exactly.
6b.   Be specific about "how" exactly.
7.   Probe for a wide range of "opportunities."
8.   A very important "enabling" question. Probe both in general and using substance of the interview.

General for interviewers

1.   We will want to hear and review the first interview for each of you.
2.   Each of you should take five nurses and five social workers.
3.   Please call any of us if there are any problems at all.
4.   Learn the questions by heart.
5.   Keep the interview to no more than a half hour (has to be closely focused throughout).

EXHIBIT 5   Major Points in the Interview Form

Date of interview _____

Person interviewed _____

Title _____

Address _____

_____

_____

1. Major points in the interview

EXHIBIT 6　Profile of Agencies and Institutions

Institution/ Agency	Type	Specialty services	Size	Location
hospital	teaching	all medical-surgical specialties, ambulatory clinics affiliate of community health centers	100s of beds	urban—large
hospital	community	all medical-surgical specialties; medical arts building adjacent; subacute units; homecare	circa 300 beds	suburban area
hospital	specialty	psychiatry—inpatient, outpatient	100s of beds	rural
hospital	generalist	all medical-surgical specialties, ambulatory care, specialty pediatric hospital part of complex	100s of beds	urban—large
community management agency		own, manage nursing homes; skilled beds and nursing facilities and assisted-living sites	own 2,181 beds and manage 1,548 beds	urban—large
community health agency– visiting nurse association with hospice unit		home health care	80 nurses 2 social workers	medium city
community health center		ambulatory care, settlement house services, specialty programs for selected persons— early intervention, etc.		urban—large
teaching hospital		all medical-surgical specialties, ambulatory care, home care	500+ beds	urban—large
community health agency— VNA		home care		urban—medium

Institution/ Agency	Type	Specialty services	Size	Location
community hospital		home care/discharge planning	200 beds	urban— medium
walk-in center		ambulatory care		urban— medium
HMO		ambulatory care, contractor for inpatient care		urban— large
multiservice agency— community		care for women, reproductive health services, residential care, transitional housing, day care for kids		urban— large
community hospital		generalist	200+ beds	urban— medium
community hospital		generalist visiting nurses association is the certified home health agency of the hospital	119 beds	urban— small
teaching hospital— specialty		women's health	200 beds	urban— medium
hospital— specialty		rehabilitation	200 beds	urban— medium

EXHIBIT 7 Profile of Participants

Participant	Position title	Highest educational preparation
Nurse # 1	vice president for patient care services	doctor of philosophy
Social worker # 1	director of social services	master's of social work
Social worker # 2	social service and discharge planning manager	master's of social work
Nurse # 2	president and chief executive officer	master's in nursing, master's of business administration
Social worker # 3	manager, geriatric social work services	master's in social work
Nurse # 3	president and chief executive officer	doctor of philosophy
Social worker # 4	director of social work	master's in social work
Nurse # 4	director of nursing	master's in nursing
Social worker # 5	president	master's in social work
Nurse # 5	vice president for subacute care	master's degree in management
Nurse # 6	clinical director	master's degree in management
Social worker # 6	staff social worker	master's degree in social work
Social worker # 6a	director of hospice, social worker	master's degree in social work
Nurse # 7	staff nurse	diploma in nursing
Social worker # 7	staff social worker	master's in social work
Social worker # 7a	staff social worker	master's in social work
Nurse # 8	vice president for nursing and nurse-in-chief	master's in nursing, doctoral—ABD (all but dissertation)
Social worker # 8	director of social service	master's of social work
Nurse # 9	president	BSN (Bachelor's of Science in Nursing), MPH (Master's in Public Health)
Social worker # 9	social worker	master's in social work
Social worker # 9	social worker	master's in social work
Nurse # 10	director of walk-in center	master's in nursing
Social worker # 10	director of social services	master's in social work
Nurse # 11	supervisor of medicine/medical specialties	bachelor's in nursing
Social worker # 11	psychiatric social work therapist	master's in social work
Nurse # 12	president and chief executive officer	doctorate
Social worker # 12	assistant director of social services	master's in social work

Participant	Position title	Highest educational preparation
Nurse # 13	vice president for nursing	master's in nursing
Social worker # 14	manager, social work department	master's in social work
Nurse/Social worker # 14	supervisor of community social work services, visiting nurses association and health services	diploma in nursing, bachelor's in adolescent development, master's in social work
Nurse # 14a	coordinator of coordinated clinical care	diploma in nursing, bachelor's in social work
Social worker # 15	clinical director	master's in social work
Nurse # 15	project director	master's in nursing
Nurse # 16	vice president of clinical services	doctorate in nursing science

EXHIBIT 8   Profile of Participants and Their Agencies

Participant	Position title	Type of institution/agency	Specialty
Nurse # 1	vice president of patient care services	teaching hospital	generalist
Social worker # 1	director of social services	teaching hospital	generalist
Social worker # 2	social service and discharge planning manager	community hospital	generalist
Nurse # 2	president and chief executive officer	community hospital	generalist
Social worker # 3	manager of geriatric social work services	specialty hospital	psychiatric
Nurse # 3	president and chief executive officer	specialty hospital	psychiatric
Social worker # 4	director of social work	teaching hospital	generalist
Nurse # 4	director of nursing	teaching hospital	generalist
Social worker # 5	president	community agency	specialist
Nurse # 5	vice president for subacute care	community agency	specialist
Nurse # 6	clinical director	community health agency, visiting nurse association	generalist
Social worker # 6	staff social worker	community health agency, visiting nurse association	generalist
Social worker # 6a	social worker and director of hospice	community health agency, visiting nurse association	hospice
Nurse # 7	registered nurse—staff	community health center	generalist
Social worker # 7	social worker—staff	community health center	generalist
Social worker # 7a	social worker—staff	community health center	generalist
Nurse # 8	vice president for nursing and nurse-in-chief	teaching hospital	generalist
Social worker # 8	director of social service	teaching hospital	generalist
Nurse # 9	president	home health, visiting nurse services	home care
Social worker # 9	social worker	home care	generalist

Participant	Position title	Type of institution/agency	Specialty
Nurse # 10	director of walk-in center	ambulatory care	generalist
Social worker # 10	director of social services	community hospital, coordination with visiting nurses association	discharge planning for home care
Nurse # 11	supervisor of medicine/medical specialties	health maintenance organization	generalist
Social worker # 11	psychiatric social worker therapist	health maintenance organization	generalist
Nurse # 12	president and chief executive officer	multiservice agency for women	specialist
Social worker # 12	assistant director of social services	multiservice agency for women	specialist
Nurse # 13	vice president for nursing	community hospital	generalist
Social worker # 14	manager of social worker department	community hospital	generalist
Nurse/Social worker # 14	supervisor of community social work services, visiting nurses association and health services	community hospital	generalist
Nurse # 14a	coordinator of coordinated clinical care	community hospital	generalist
Social worker # 15	clinical director of project for pregnant women using substances	specialty hospital	specialty—women's health
Nurse # 15	project director of a pregnancy and substance abuse project	specialty hospital	specialty—women's health
Nurse # 16	vice president of clinical services	specialty hospital	specialty—rehabilitation

EXHIBIT 9   Consent Form for Survey Participants

I have agreed to participate in this study and understand that responses may be used anonymously in a forthcoming book, *Managed Care: Social Work and Nursing Uniting to Take Charge in the Community. A Model of Collaboration, Coordination, and Accountability*, by Joellen W. Hawkins, Carole W. Pearce, and Nancy W. Veeder.

Name _____

Title _____

Date Interview Completed _____

EXHIBIT 10   Themes from the Interviews

EVOLUTION OF COLLABORATION

expectation of collaboration
taught to be cooperative, not competitive in socialization to agency
share issues in common and work on them together
leadership in nursing and social work agreed to collaborate
not power play about control but patients have needs
one of first hospitals to go with nurse/social worker team approach (almost 15 years ago)
nurses, social workers, and physicians work together in triad in inpatient, subacute,
     homecare, community
more divergence with diagnostic related groups
different orientations but some similar core
model has always been there—not sure how collaborative or effective it has been
worked out social contracts with each other, how to treat each other and with patients
     and their families (psychiatric mental health setting) versus a pecking order with
     physician at top (as in some places)
partnership in community centers
depended on each other in early days
history of nursing being a closed system, alienated social workers, misuse of power in
     nursing; identity with the aggressor—taking power for its own sake; few role models
     for nursing; under siege—got kicked—kicked other departments; long strained
     relationship; parallel = not working together; poor role clarification; no sense of
     collaboration; some positive examples in specialties, e.g., AIDS group practice,
     pediatrics, hematology/oncology multidisciplinary team
traditional within traditional roles; enrichment with clinical people—put premium on
     quality and quality care
nurturing role of leaders sets tone of collaboration and teamwork
always been multidisciplinary team in long-term care dictated by regulations
very large nurse to social worker ratio so collaboration small part of agency; nurse
     must be involved in case before social worker needed; usually three to four disci-
     plines involved at that point
history of collaboration from history of agency, not hierarchical
interacting since the 1920s; on discharge planning for 20–25 years
always been there
12 years of collaboration; work closely together
over 100 year history of collaboration
collaboration in case management—now case management department bigger than
     social work ever was and head is a social worker
primarily in external system—discharge planning, aftercare phase, long-term care
5 years ago began case management; social workers and nurses have always been
     collaborative now true collaborators
comanagement of a project between social work and nursing—designed that way

PLUSES

combines collective talents
needs of each patient

hold to what it is that patient needs then look at what each can contribute and where overlaps are

what can we do as a team to aid patients

gray areas allow for flexibility

no turf situations

two very different types of training—way it comes together—ideal model

interdependent on one another; one can't exist without other in continuity of care

both have different orientations, offer different angles on same issue

social workers see whole picture, nurses (especially ADN [associate degree in nursing]) task oriented, not see picture outside institution

working together focus on the here and now—what can we do here and what will happen later

more mature and secure professionals—less oriented toward power, begin to relate to body of knowledge and more conceptually with health care delivery systems

more autonomous the parties, more collaboration and more respect for each other

patient centered care—what they need; nurse brings pathophysiology understanding; social workers synapse with patient about what patient is going through, understand how to cope with things

complement each other

social worker brings support and facilitates the next dimension of care; keeps people on a continuum

increased ability to have autonomy

social work role in helping staff with interpersonal relations within facility; serve as consultant around nursing interpersonal problems

only reach goal of someone going home at highest level with a team; nurses get patient up to highest possible level, social workers make sure home environment is ready

best job in shortest time—social workers have knowledge nurses don't and can deal with those issues efficiently

help each other, share case conferences; consultation, collaboration, communication

holistic approach to care, support each other, take more time with patients

each brings unique perspective

appreciative acknowledgement of each other's work

impediment to patient's recovery—social worker is adjunct to focus on impediment, facilitate recovery with the nurse

rally forces with patient in crisis to get patients home

both look at whole family through two sets of eyes

evaluate physical theory, clinical care, social aspects of care, give missing parts of the puzzle

primary motivation is patient's benefit; social workers are patient advocates, deal with psychosocial issues; nurses deal more with medical concerns

both advocates for patient; see beyond medical needs

nurses in front line working with physicians, seeing patients; will call and refer to social workers

social workers know external community best

combination of two world views dynamite

social work in hospital setting had much more collegial role with physicians than did nurses

partnership of social workers and nurses in acute care has allowed social workers to provide the broader perspective because nurses in acute care have not been as connected to the community

focus on better client care and not on professional self-image

complement each other—should not ask person to be physically and psychically undefended at the same time; nurses can do one and social workers the other

holistic approach; a "natural collaboration"; "the best of both worlds"—people with training in emotional and mental health and people with training in physical health; social work helps nursing understand human behavior better as nurses want a quick fix; social work helps nursing realize we can't always cause a change directly

nurses aware of so many social issues that surround patient and family and no time to reach out and contact community resources; in working together needs can be met

MINUSES

fabulous practitioners need business types too

skill development needed to be full partners

conflicts with other members of team—physicians, psychologists, especially in psychiatric mental health

not always perfectly clear boundaries; example social worker contacting visiting nurses association re: discharge planning

best worked out by team and not a directive

pay differentials between social work and nursing

nurses on three 8-hour shifts; social workers 9–5 M through F; no weekend coverage

no electronic record keeping = complex communications

communication needs to be crystal clear

difference in education—frustrating for social worker: 2 versus 6 years of preparation; different with bachelor's and master's degreed nurses

frustration of social work—role in health care changes—duplication of what nurses do

frustration of no tangible task to do (social worker) versus nurse

nurses could shut out social worker with lingo

nursing's self-esteem more fragile

social work well grounded conceptually but not always operationalize

turf; see patients as segmented and not as a whole

resistance to bringing social workers into community and to psychiatric nurses in the community

underpinnings of two lesser professions in eyes of others still there (social work and nursing)

inherent in delivery system—does not always support social work—get rid of social workers

length of stay for patients

need to look at where we pull apart and where we pull together

forced to change because of money and it doesn't feel good

some nurses resistant to change and want control

cultural change as go up acuity level they are administering

resources scarce

problems with nurses as case managers and leaders of team; social work becomes more fuzzy

barriers to keep us from doing each other's jobs

difficulties in communication

high anxiety about the future

competition in face of job security, ambiguity

social workers feel like low person on hierarchy in hospital

disparity in salaries, number of social workers

question of philosophical match

logistical difficulties, lack of face-to-face interactions

lack of common language, lack of understanding of macro health issues

nurses lack understanding of cultural issues, unfriendly to persons of different cultures

social workers better than nurses with persons with HIV

deciding who is most appropriate person for each role—e.g., case manager

fear of losing status if nursing was in control of managed care system in and out of hospital

nurses uncomfortable with ambiguity—see things as black and white; social workers see things as gray

nurses try to do everything—be rescuers

nurses need to make transition of locus of control when in the community—who is really in charge—the client!

creative tension between the two professions; cultures within the professions; conflicts around when to let clients do for themselves; how much to be directly involved in clients' problems; nurses may feel social workers aren't doing their job because the problems aren't fixed; nurses tend to be reactive, social workers trained to be nonreactive

problems when one steps on the other's toes or one discipline becomes territorial

OUTCOMES

where patients go after discharge

can patients care for selves

readmissions

patient satisfaction with services

other consumers such as families

how successful triaging is

what is reimbursed for

patient functioning—able to do activities of daily living, go back to work, etc.

patient satisfaction such as being on time, etc.

look at health not disease

satisfy what patients need by their definitions

managed care—who is least expensive provider

customer service satisfaction
avoiding emergency room visits
is patient in stable social system environment
readmits to acute care
length of stay inpatient
days patient was denied for placement—social work or nursing variables contributing
    to that?
social work not available for weekend discharge?
need to work together to come up with measurement including psychological outcomes
define what we are trying to achieve—work with clients as to what they want to achieve,
    how to get those results
infection rate, return to hospital, patient satisfaction, functional ability, pain manage-
    ment, school attendance
care maps—critical pathways
efficiency issues
infection rate, deep vein thrombosis, comorbidities
pain scales—subjective measure
developmental milestones
prenatal outcomes
goals take time to achieve in social work—not a product
evaluate together and not attribute outcomes to any one profession or group
physician satisfaction with outcomes of programs
behavioral change in patient
profile high-risk profile patients—then target for in-depth interface work
in model for pregnant women using drugs—evaluated pregnancy outcomes, stopping
    substance use or not
more in terms of nurses versus social workers—we need literature on what we are
    doing—expected outcomes

DIRECT ACCESS BY PATIENTS TO HEALTH CARE PROVIDERS

voucher system—employee can access provider chosen
most physicians not capable of managing social aspects of care
physicians as gatekeepers will keep us out
see changes with partnerships between nurses and social workers
work together to recommend services
lots of untapped opportunities under managed care
orders written by whom: payer justifies need for service and not by whom
service tied more to reimbursement and less to provider system
capitation: keep more money if keep patient well
collaborate with physicians on telephone calls to patients; break from 50-minute visit
    model to shorter visits in psychiatric mental health to see how people are doing
optimism; experiences have been positive
primary care is difficult role (nurse practitioner)—often can't refer due to cost
best and most cost effective care may not be physician—payment structure needs
    to change

access getting harder

incentive to do less today

through physician as gatekeeper and home intake from physician; direct access for patients to home care services

health maintenance organization gives access, tools for home care

demand by patient—greater role in care

yes more access—"one stop shopping in health care"—especially for high-risk clients

not more—managed care companies will control whom we access and how

IDEAL SYSTEM OF COLLABORATION BETWEEN NURSES AND SOCIAL WORKERS

social workers and registered nurses direct carriers of services

go direct nurse practitioners—triage

social workers, registered nurses establish primary care practices

pediatrics and ob/gyn primary care model with nurse practitioners and social workers

focus on patient need instead of what I am trained to do

who is best equipped to do what for patient

coordinated care program to keep frail elders at home—social workers and nurses

case manager—best person for need of patient at a point in time; could change with patient's needs

note: no one wants to be a case and no one wants to be managed

who offers skill needed based on assessment of patients, activities of daily living, etc.

refer persons into services and keep people away through prevention

goal—keep people out of acute care

more case management beyond hospital and on a continuum

case management of a broad community of patients

settlement model as ideal

work together in schools—social workers and nurses

continuum of care

share burden of responsibility for patient (such as a suicidal patient)

need to get back to values; examine what are our values

nurses to run long-term care facilities; why not other facilities

home care—roles across the continuum; act as resource coordinators

coordination among settings—a circle of care

case managers as physician extenders—protect quality and access to care

consider food and transportation for elders, housing and social concerns—consolidate these and health care needs

work with physicians to establish referral system

connect directly with patients

establish bridge programs: nurse could visit patients in home, set up a program of care, find people who need us

community health center—ideal setting to offer all services to family in one setting

social work and nursing have one department and not two

early interventions for new families postpartum

advanced practice nurse and social worker model for collaboration
a true interdisciplinary team; both go on home visits; all health care needs met at one
    site; setting should be dignified; separate women's services from men's
team system

a. Prevention

federal government moving toward a medical model
need collaborative system to get together and disperse as needed
information system online—not repeat information
move into community more
collaborate with managed care systems—one requested social worker on each of
    their patients
manage people in workplace, home, manage stress to keep them well
computer access for elders through telephone-monitor elderly, keep in touch through
    cable television
reimbursement for phone calls by providers—prevent emergency room visits, inpatient
    stays—experiment in psychiatry now; check in with patients, crisis management
    over the phone to allay crisis
center in schools with social workers and nurses working together on preventive model
collaborate as case managers: work in welfare system, school system, out in community
social workers and nurses work together to come up with pragmatic ways for early
    intervention
rotate nurses from inpatient to outpatient; collaborate in outpatient
care should be patient; more emphasis in community care
models like Head Start
need diversity to reach patients and cultural sensitivity
managed care inhibits this—not an altruistic system; at their agency strong health
    promotion focus; need to negotiate with managed care companies

b. Complementary Systems

patients fearful to tell providers of use
National Institutes of Health Mind Body Institute
need champions in medicine to give credibility
question of do complementary therapies find a home in the health professions?
how to measure outcomes?
must mix Eastern and Western to meet needs of patients
conservative community—patients don't ask about other therapies
question of mind and body balance
look at how what is going on makes person feel; anything that helps as long as it is
    not in conflict
need to do empirical studies to show what works
bring in as adjunct to (Western medicine) treatment
take care so people don't get victimized

need to work with healers for better health care—nurses and social workers can facilitate process

payment for this care a problem

need to incorporate Eastern philosophy of healing with Western view—be open to it

have alternative healers in place within the health maintenance organization

very important in helping persons with substance abuse problems: acupuncture, spiritual healers, therapeutic touch, stress management, relaxation, nutrition, vitamin supplements; best approach in substance abuse is not medical approach

not more involvement—we don't know what the outcomes are—a hard sell with managed care companies

OPPORTUNITIES

registered nurses and social workers be entrepreneurs

establish private practices

hire physicians as needed

professional organizations join forces

social workers, nurses work in large group practices with physicians; serve as case managers to keep people out of hospitals or move them in and out quickly

social workers work in big group practices; collaborate on intensive cases (models now in psych at this setting)—social workers, nurses, physicians

social workers and nurses embrace the power they have together

see patients and families together in the community to talk about goals together

oncology, hospice care—advocate for patients with physicians so social network can absorb needs; nurses can predict trajectory across the continuum; help plan in home and for future admissions, etc.

primary care—run clinics and centers, use physicians for referrals

social workers and nurses could be unbelievable team in the managed care market

locate out in the community—too expensive in hospital

behavioral and mental health facilities

school based programs, long-term care, elderly , subacute care

whole disease management

screening in community—as in grocery stores

get in on capitation

be culturally competent and educate community; act as liaisons between Western medicine and immigrant healing practices

create patient learning center

stop reeling under managed care and begin to say "let's all take charge"

forced collaboration under managed care; equal opportunities for both professions under managed care for social workers and nurses

look at outcomes—be introspective—critical evaluation of what we do and why

EXAMPLES

housing for elderly at Massachusetts General Hospital—social worker and nurse teams

outreach to health centers that are not freestanding—contract with these for services

executive health programs
domestic violence, drugs, alcohol, smoking—take lead in models
school based clinics, women's centers, daycare
Tucson model
D. Brooten et al.'s work
colorectal screening—at grocery store along with coupon for high fiber foods
domestic violence, terminal illness

OTHER ISSUES

how to keep each profession sharp so they don't become enmeshed and mediocre—stay
   on cutting edge
reinforce in education that working together is important and that care(ing) is important
use models from social work of supervision in nursing
look at career plans of the members of the unit
problems of gender dynamics in nursing and in social work
most case management learned through continuing education not organized in academia
hard to move ahead in New England—deeply rooted
traditional social work roles are gone; social work education needs to prepare for today's
   world; harder to develop roles if not taught
most nurses don't know what is going on
pay attention to spiritual needs of clients
need more education for professionals about managed care
compensate both better in managed care
educate both professions together
revamp both social work and nursing education—set stage for how people go out in
   the world
education too rigid especially social work
focus on wellness and health
keep people out of hospital
look at alternative modalities
be proactive not reactive
provide quality care at a lower cost
social workers have to be aggressive as a profession—social work has a problem with
   aggression—usually passive and insecure

EXHIBIT 11   Participants in Study

Susan S. Bailis, MSW
Shelley L. Baranowski, RN, MS
Evelyn E. Bonander, ACSW
Don Bowdoin, LICSW
Joyce C. Clifford, RN, MSN, FAAN
Jeanette G. Clough, MS, MHA
Amba Coltman, BCSW, LICSW
Pamela Duchene, DNSc, RN
Nancy A. Dineen, RN, MSN
Marybeth Duffy, MSW, LICSW
Anna C. Foster, RN, BSW
Janice L. Gibeau, RN, Ph.D., CS
Phebe Goldman, RN, BSN, MPH
Jack Haynes, MSW, LICSW
Kathleen Kinneen, MSW, MBA, LICSW
Barbara Kotz, MSW, LICSW
Kathy MacDonald, LICSW
Joyce Marshall, RN
Noreen G. Mattis, RN, M.Ed.
Jane B. Mayer, MSW, LICSW
Susan A. Myers, MSW, LICSW
Caralyn Nash, LICSW
Kathleen M. Orr, MSW, CCM
Patricia Palermo, MS, RN
Ellen Parker, MSW
Elizabeth Reilinger, Ph.D.
Jean Robbins, LICSW, CDP
Joyce McDonald Shannon, RN, MS
Irene Sommers, BSN, MBA
Linda A. Souza, BSN
Sheila Upchurch, MSW
Gail Kuhn Weissman, RN, Ed.D., FAAN
Susan Lacey Williams, RN, MSW, LICSW

Index

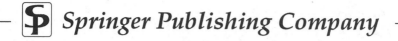

Springer Publishing Company

Geriatric Home Health Care
The Collaboration of Physicians, Nurses, and Social Workers

Philip W. Brickner, MD, **F. Russell Kellogg**, MD,
Anthony J. Lechich, MD, **Roberta Lipsman**, MSSW,
Linda K. Scharer, MUP, Editors

Drawing on more than 20 years of work in geriatric home health care, the editors of this book share their experiences in creating and managing home care programs for the frail aged. They have compiled information from diverse disciplines, including medicine, nursing, gerontology, and social services. In addition to in-depth coverage of important clinical issues such as functional ability, mental health, and disease and accident prevention, the book focuses on critical programmatic issues including:

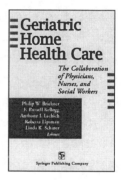

- the use of professional physician, nurse, and social worker teams
- paraprofessional and family supports
- ethical issues and strategies about making choices in life support decisions
- methods for bringing students into this field of care

Furthermore, the editors include analyses of four long-term home health care programs, each with a substantial history of success in working through administrative, financial, and bureaucratic problems. This book should be required reading for all health professionals working with the elderly in long-term home health care settings.

1996   320pp   0-8261-9450-8   hardcover

536 Broadway, New York, NY 10012-3955 • (212) 431-4370 • Fax (212) 941-7842

ℙ *Springer Publishing Company*

Planning, Implementing, and Evaluating Critical Pathways
A Guide for Health Care Survival into the 21st Century

Patricia C. Dykes, MA, RN
Kathleen Wheeler, PhD, CS, APRN, Editors
Foreword by **Karen Zander,** RN, MS, CS, FAAN

This is a practical guide to developing critical pathways for a multitude of settings — acute care, ambulatory, home care, rehabilitation, and long-term care. The book takes the reader from the very first steps of critical pathway design, through the ins- and-outs of implementation, and then assists the reader with evaluating patient and systems outcomes and improving practice. Concrete examples are given of how to adapt pathways to meet the needs of individual institutions and how to incorporate them into a continuous quality improvement process. Specific legal concerns are addressed in a chapter by attorneys who are also nurses; and an entire chapter is devoted to the computerization of pathways. Students, educators, administrators and clinicians will find this an essential resource for providing quality care, efficient case management, and a sound outcomes management program.

Contents:

An Introduction to Critical Pathways • Designing and Implementing Critical Pathways: An Overview • Copathways and Algorithms • Data Collection, Outcomes Measurement and Variance Analysis • Critical Pathways in the Acute Care Setting • Critical Pathways in Ambulatory Care • Critical Pathways in Home Care: Developing a Psychiatric Home Care Program • Critical Pathways in Rehabilitation and Long-Term Care • Liability Issues in Development, Implementation and Documentation of Critical Pathways • Critical Pathways and Computerization: Issues Driving the Need for Automation

1997   182pp   0-8261-9790-6   hardcover

536 Broadway, New York, NY 10012-3955 • (212) 431-4370 • Fax (212) 941-7842

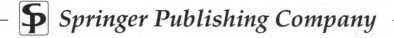

S *Springer Publishing Company*

Measurement Tools in Patient Education

Barbara K. Redman, PhD, RN

This book draws together instruments for measuring outcomes in patient education from a wide variety of sources. Fifty-two actual tools are included. Each tool is accompanied by a descriptive review, a critique, and information on administration, scoring, and psychometric properties.

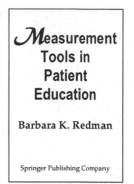

Measurement Tools in Patient Education

Barbara K. Redman

Springer Publishing Company

Particular attention is given to the different cultures in which the instrument has been used. Two introductory chapters give a basic orientation to the field. Designed for nurses and other health professionals involved in patient education.

Contents:

Part I: An Introduction
- Measurement in Patient Education Practice and Research
- Measurement of Self-Efficacy and Quality of Life in Patient Education

Part II. Description of Tools
- Basic Patient Education Needs
- Diabetes
- Arthritis
- Asthma
- Pregnancy, Childbirth, and Parenting
- Other Clinical Topics
- Health Promotion, Disease Prevention and Increasing Quality of Life
- Appendix: Summary of Tools

1997 408pp 0-8261-9860-0 softcover

536 Broadway, New York, NY 10012-3955 • (212) 431-4370 • Fax (212) 941-7842

S *Springer Publishing Company*

Chronic Illness and the Older Adult
Advances in Gerontological Nursing

Elizabeth A. Swanson, PhD, RN
Toni Tripp-Reimer, PhD, RN, FAAN, Editors

This volume addresses the problem of chronic illness in the elderly. It gives an excellent overview of the issues, followed by insightful chapters on physical and psychosocial issues and nursing management. Topics discussed include health promotion, care in the community, the impact of ethnicity on chronic illness, pain, social isolation, and qualitative research. Contributers include Juliet Corbin, Joanne Sabol Stevenson, and Janice Morse. Nursing students will find this a valuable introduction to the topic, and practicing nurses will find in-depth current information on issues of importance to them.

Contents: Chronic Illness Issues and the Older Adult, *Margaret Dimond, Marci Catanzaro and Margarethe Lorensen* • Health Promotion for Chronically Ill Elders, *Joanne Sabol Stevenson* • Caring for the Aged in the Community, *Juliet M. Corbin and Julie C. Cherry* • Chronic Pain in the Elderly, *Keela A. Herr and Paula R. Mobily* • Ethnicity, Aging, and Chronic Illness, *Toni Tripp-Reimer* •Social Support, Social Networks, and the Problem of Loneliness in Elder Care, *Bethel Ann Powers* • Qualitative Research and Chronic Illness, *Janice M. Morse and Cheryl A. Dellasega* • Nursing Homes and the Chronically Ill Resident: Policy and Issues, *Marilyn J. Rantz and Mary Zwygart-Stauffacher* • Epilogue: Policy Issues Related to Accessible Health Care for Older Adults, *Elizabeth A. Swanson*

1997   234pp   0-8261-9111-8   hardcover

536 Broadway, New York, NY 10012-3955 • (212) 431-4370 • Fax (212) 941-7842